Unspoken
The Unbearable Weight of Infertility
Cheryl Dowling

Finesse Literary Press Ltd.

First edition 2025 published by Finesse Literary Press Ltd.

Finesse

Contents

Dedication   1

Introduction   2

1. IVF Warrior   15

2. The Infertility Rollercoaster   29

3. Why Didn't Anyone Tell Me   37

4. Fertility Confessions   48

5. The Waiting Game   62

6. When Infertility Tests Everything   70

7. The Mental Toll   85

8. Grief Runs Deep   97

9. Your Voice Matters   109

10. The Club We Never Wanted To Join   117

Conclusion   126

Dear Warrior: Words for the Moments That   133
Feel Impossible

Acknowledgements   150

To anyone who has felt the unique pain and challenges of infertility. To those who have fought battles that most will never see or understand. And to the ones who, for far too long, have felt alone in the struggle.

This book is for you.

May you find comfort in knowing that the silent thoughts, feelings, and struggles you have faced do not make you broken; they make you human. May these words bring light to the darkness of this chapter in your life, reminding you that even in the shadows, you are never alone.

Introduction

Infertility doesn't just touch one part of your life. It takes over everything. It follows you into every conversation, every decision, every quiet moment. It turns life into an unbearable waiting game.

It's the gut punch of another pregnancy announcement, the sting of a well-meaning but painful comment from someone who doesn't understand. The silent grief of watching another month slip away. It's feeling disconnected from your own body—as if it has betrayed you in ways you never thought possible.

It is friendships shifting as conversations become harder to join and relationships being tested under the weight of stress, grief, and unanswered questions. It's the overwhelming ache of feeling stuck while the rest of the world moves forward without you.

It's avoiding certain aisles, conversations, and events because the weight of it is too much.

It's a holiday gathering where someone casually asks, *So when are you having kids?* In that moment, you try so hard not to let the emotions overtake you. They don't know; they don't understand what it's like to be here, to want something so deeply and feel like it's always just out of reach.

Infertility is waking up every morning with the same aching question: *When will it be my turn?* And trying to fall asleep every night with the same unrelenting fear: *What if it never is?*

It's spending what feels like an eternity inside clinic walls, sitting in silent waiting rooms where no one makes eye contact. It's steadying your breath, trying to push past the tightness in your chest, bracing for the uncertainty of what this next appointment will bring.

It's stepping outside the clinic walls into a world that remains unchanged while yours has just fallen apart. You are standing there, frozen, not knowing where to go or what to do next. You wonder: how will you move forward when everything inside you is breaking?

Infertility is that moment. The moment when the rest of the world keeps moving forward, but you are stuck in this place. It's the loneliness of feeling like no one else notices.

And then, you receive the dreaded phone calls. The nurse's voice—gentle but detached—confirms what you already knew in your heart. *Another failed cycle. Another step further from the life you so desperately want.*

Infertility is silent grief. It is learning to carry a pain that others don't recognize. It is showing up to work after getting devastating news. It's forcing a smile or congratulations while your heart breaks. It's pretending to be okay when inside, you're barely holding it together.

A Defining Moment

I never expected infertility to be part of my story, let alone define so much of my life. And yet, through the struggle, heartbreak, and uncertainty, I found something I never anticipated: a community and a place where I wasn't alone in my grief, my frustration, or my hope.

When I first started sharing my story on The IVF Warrior, I hesitated. I wasn't sure if my voice mattered. I wasn't sure if I had the right words. But I knew one thing: I was tired of feeling alone. I was searching for connection, for someone—anyone—who understood the depths of what I was going through and could say, *Me too. I know how this feels.*

So I typed out a post, hit "share," and held my breath.

What I never expected was the flood of responses. Messages from people who had been carrying this pain in silence, who had never spoken about it out loud, who finally felt seen for the first time. I heard from others who had been carrying the same grief, the same fears, the same exhaustion.

I read stories of failed transfers, years of waiting, failed relationships, and impossible decisions. I read stories from people who had been fighting for years, who had run out of finances and options, who were still trying to find hope. And in those stories, I saw pieces of my own story. I realized then that I wasn't just telling my story; I was telling *our* story.

Suddenly, I wasn't just speaking for myself anymore. I had unknowingly become part of something bigger, a movement, a community, a space for those who had spent too long suffering in silence. And through those conversations, I realized just how desperately this space was needed.

Who I Am & Why This Book Exists

I've been through nine IVF cycles, multiple losses, endless injections, surgeries, failed transfers, and the soul-crushing experience of watching my dream drift further away with each passing year. At my lowest, I turned to social media, searching for someone who could put into words what I was feeling. When I didn't find that space, I created it. I started The IVF Warrior as a way to connect, process, and let others know they weren't alone.

But my understanding of this pain didn't begin with my own journey. Before I ever walked this path, I sat across from countless women in pain, women who shared their stories of infertility, loss, and grief with me in counseling sessions. I ran support groups, created self-care programs, and worked with those who felt like they had nowhere else to turn.

I listened to women try to put the trauma of their losses into words, to explain the turmoil of infertility, and transcend the loneliness that no one else seemed to understand fully. I heard their desperation, their exhaustion, their longing for an escape from the relentless pain. Some would say they wanted to feel numb, to stop feeling so deeply because the weight of it all was too much to bear.

I worked as an intake counselor, speaking with thousands of individuals every month. People who called in were raw with emotion and simply needed someone, anyone, to listen. I heard the hesitation in their voices, the heartbreak in their words as they explained they had infertility and didn't know where to turn. Many were seeking validation; others just wanted to say the words out loud to someone who wouldn't minimize or dismiss their pain.

At the time, I could deeply empathize—but I didn't truly understand. I didn't know that one day, I would be on the other end of that phone call, needing the very same space to be heard. Everything I had witnessed, the suffering, the frustration, the profound grief, would become my reality. And when it did, I finally understood the weight of it in a way I never could have before.

That experience shaped the way I now approach infertility, loss, and mental health. It made me want to change the conversation and ensure that no one going through this ever feels as alone as so many of the women I once spoke with.

For too long, mental health and infertility have been treated as separate struggles—mental health discussed in whispers, infertility ignored altogether. But infertility isn't just physical; it's emotional, psychological, and deeply intertwined. And yet, too often, it is ignored.

The anxiety. The depression. The way it makes you question your own worth, your identity, your place in the world. The way it isolates you, even from those who love you most.

I have seen firsthand how infertility and loss impact every part of a person's well-being. It's not just about the cycles, the medications, or the procedures. It's about the emotional devastation of watching time slip away, the exhaustion of hoping when hope feels impossible, and the grief of mourning something that others don't even recognize as a loss.

For too long, these experiences have been brushed aside and treated as an unfortunate part of the process instead of the life-altering trauma that they truly are. But they deserve to be acknowledged. The pain is real. The heartbreak is real. And the need for support is urgent.

That's why I started speaking up. I continue to advocate every day because no one should suffer in silence. No one should feel like their pain is invisible. Infertility is hard enough without the added weight of feeling alone.

Through my work, my advocacy, and now this book, my mission is simple: to ensure that no one navigating infertility ever has to feel like they are carrying this alone.

If you have ever felt unheard, overlooked, or dismissed in this journey, know that I see you. I hear you. And I will continue to fight to make sure that the world hears you too.

I know how painful and exhausting this journey can be. I've walked this path, and I know the endless nights spent crying in the dark, the ache of wanting something so profoundly, and feeling like it's *always just out of reach*. I understand how infertility consumes your thoughts, your body, and your identity, reshaping who you are.

That's why I wrote this book.

To be the voice I needed most when I first started this journey.

To give the words that feel impossible to say out loud.

To validate what you're feeling and remind you that everything you're going through is real—and it matters.

Infertility is isolating. It's the kind of pain that often goes unspoken, leaving those struggling feeling unseen and misunderstood. There is also a lack of honest resources for those facing infertility. Too often, conversations are clinical and detached, ignoring the emotional weight of every setback, every failed cycle, every loss. I needed to change that.

This book exists because infertility is more than a diagnosis. It's a battle that changes you. It forces you to navigate grief while still holding onto hope, a balance that feels nearly impossible at times.

It's heartbreak and resilience.

It's feeling like the world is moving forward while you're standing still.

It's knowing the pain is real but feeling like no one sees it.

I wrote this book so you wouldn't have to carry this alone. Your pain is valid. Your story matters. And no matter what happens next, you are not alone.

What This Book Is and What It's Not

This book is not a step-by-step guide to fertility treatments. It won't promise you a happy ending because I know firsthand that this journey is unpredictable.

What I can offer, however, is honesty—a raw, unfiltered look at the realities of infertility, the lessons I've learned, and the strength I found in the midst of it all.

This book is the voice I wish I had when I was drowning in uncertainty. It's the words I needed when I was crying on my bathroom floor after another failed cycle, when I was consumed by *what-ifs*, feeling like I was yelling into a void and no one was listening.

It's the reminder that your pain is real, your grief is valid, and you are not alone in this.

I want this book to be a source of empowerment. Infertility has a way of making you feel powerless—as if your body is betraying you. But you are not powerless. You hold so much power in your choices, in your voice, and in the way you advocate for yourself.

But more than anything, this book is a conversation. It represents a place where we can sit together in the hard moments, where we can hold space for each other and remember that even in our darkest moments, we are not alone.

Throughout these pages, we will talk about the emotional toll of infertility, the grief, the anger, the exhaustion, and the unspoken challenges. We'll talk about the mental weight of constantly living in the unknown, the anxiety of waiting, and the fear of getting your hopes up. We'll talk about relationships, the friendships that shift, the family dynamics that change, and the strain this puts on even the strongest marriages.

We will talk about trauma—about how infertility leaves scars even after the treatments end. Because the truth is, no matter how this journey unfolds, infertility stays with you. And we need to talk about that too. It changes the way you see yourself, how you navigate joy and grief, and how you react to life's uncertainties.

The scars remain. The years of waiting don't vanish. The trauma doesn't erase itself overnight.

You'll carry the memories of every failed cycle, every heartbreak, every impossible decision. You'll still flinch at certain questions and unexpectedly feel the weight of the grief that once consumed you.

This book is about acknowledging the emotional wreckage that infertility leaves behind. It's about piecing yourself back together after loss, after heartbreak, after years of waiting. It's about rediscovering who you are beyond this struggle, beyond the pain, beyond the uncertainty.

And in that, there is also hope.

Because even in the depths of infertility, even in the moments when hope feels impossible, it still exists. Hope in finding support, in making informed choices, and hope in knowing that, no matter how your story unfolds, you are more than infertility.

If You've Ever Felt Alone, This Book Is for You

This book is for the one searching for answers, for comfort, for a sense of belonging in a world that often overlooks this struggle. For the one who feels invisible, unheard, and weighed down by the loneliness of this journey.

For the one drowning in uncertainty, consumed by an endless storm of thoughts and emotions, wondering if the heartbreak will ever subside.

For the one questioning if they're strong enough to keep going...if their heart can handle one more disappointment...if hope is still worth holding onto.

And for the one who made it to the other side but carries the weight of everything it took to get there, I see you. I know that every step, every sacrifice, and every heartbreak still lingers.

If you are in this place right now, hear me when I say this: you are not alone.

I know how much this hurts. I know how hard it is to hold onto hope when everything feels impossible. I know what it's like to question if you can keep going, if you are *strong* enough to survive another heartbreak. And I know what it's like to carry the weight of impossible decisions and unbearable grief.

So if you are reading this and feeling like no one understands, please hear me: I do.

I see you.

I know how much this hurts.

I know what it's like to feel invisible, forgotten in your pain.

But I also know your story is not over. And no matter what happens next, you won't face it alone.

So take a deep breath, turn the page, and know this: You are seen. You are heard. And what you feel, every ounce of it, matters.

Chapter One

IVF Warrior

I never thought infertility would be part of my story. I hadn't prepared for or even thought much about it. Infertility was never openly discussed in school, among friends, or in the media in a way that actually depicted it or reflected its actual emotional weight. I never knew how common it was, who was at risk, or how deeply it could impact every aspect of one's life.

Infertility is rarely talked about, making it even more terrifying when it happens to you.

Do you remember being young, dreaming about the future? What your life would look like, the must-haves, the hopes, the dreams? For me, motherhood was always part of that dream. There were many things I was unsure of in life, but one thing I never doubted was that one day, I would be a mom. It was something I felt deep within my soul.

Before infertility, I planned baby names and imagined nursery colors. I thought about the milestones, the ultrasound pictures on the fridge, the moment I'd get to see two pink lines. I never once considered the possibility that getting pregnant wouldn't just happen. That I'd have to *fight for it.*

Ignorance is bliss when it comes to fertility. Like so many, I never thought I'd be part of this statistic. I never imagined the reality I would one day face.

The First Signs Something Was Wrong

At first, I wasn't worried. I knew it could take some time, but the negative tests piled up month after month. I told myself it was normal. I reassured myself that the next month would be different. But as time passed, worry crept in.

The day I finally scheduled a doctor's appointment, I still had hope. I believed I'd walk out with a simple solution. Maybe I just needed to time things better or take a pill to regulate my cycles.

My gynecologist reassured me that I was *young* and *healthy*, prescribed six months of medication, and casually suggested losing some weight because of my polycystic ovary syndrome (PCOS). She told me I'd be pregnant in no time.

Six months.

Six negative pregnancy tests.

Six times, my heart broke.

I still remember how my hope slowly faded, month after month.

The Test That Changed Everything

When my doctor finally ordered more tests, I felt relieved. At least I was doing something. But nothing could have prepared me for the results.

What started as a routine fertility test to check my fallopian tubes and uterus turned into a nightmare I couldn't wake up from. The pain from the test was shocking and unexpected, but the results were even worse.

The clinician's face was unreadable as he studied the screen. When he finally spoke, his words made my stomach drop.

Both of my fallopian tubes were blocked, damaged, and completely unusable. My uterus wasn't shaped the way it should be.

What followed was an appointment with my fertility doctor to confirm what we already suspected. Without IVF, I had a zero percent chance of conceiving.

The moment you hear the words you have infertility or need treatments like IVF, time freezes. Everything you thought you knew about your future shifts, and suddenly, you're navigating an unfamiliar and overwhelming reality. It's a moment no one prepares you for.

The moment I heard the words: *IVF is your only option*, my life changed forever.

Processing the Reality of Infertility

I walked out of the clinic in a daze. The world outside was painfully normal; cars passed by and people walked down the sidewalk, completely unaware that my entire life had just shifted in a way I wasn't prepared for. My legs felt unsteady, my breath shallow, my thoughts racing.

I wasn't just leaving an appointment. I was leaving behind the life I thought I'd have. My entire future changed in a matter of moments, and I had no idea how to process it.

Suddenly, I was thrown into a world I never imagined, one filled with appointments, injections, and protocols.

When I sat across from my fertility specialist, listening to every detail of what IVF entailed, I felt like I was drowning. The terminology was overwhelming. The cost was terrifying. The uncertainty was suffocating.

Why me? What did I do to deserve this? They can't be right. Complete shock, disbelief, and panic hit all at once. The heaviness was paralyzing.

Questions, realizations, doubts, and fears crashed into my mind.

Could we even afford IVF?

And finally, the most heartbreaking thought of all: *What if I never become a mom?* The person who walked into that appointment was not the same person who walked out of it.

Overwhelmed and Unprepared

My journey was filled with more obstacles than I ever could have imagined. It wasn't just one diagnosis or one hurdle to overcome; it was layer after layer of complications, each one making the dream of having a baby feel further out of reach.

I have endometriosis and PCOS, conditions that have caused me pain for years but were never fully explained to me in terms of what they could mean for my fertility. I have a septate and bicornuate uterus—words I had never heard but would soon come to understand all too well. I learned that both of my fallopian tubes were completely blocked, meaning there was no chance of conceiving without *a lot* of help.

I endured seven laparoscopies, each one a reminder that my body wasn't working the way it was supposed to. I had a salpingectomy to remove my damaged tubes and a hysteroscopic metroplasty to help reshape my uterus. Each procedure was another piece of hope, another attempt to fix what felt so painfully broken.

But the hardest surgery of all was the one that took something from me: the salpingectomy. The day I lost my fallopian tubes.

I had spent years believing that my body could do this, that I just needed time, the proper medications, and the right doctor. But when they told me my tubes were too damaged and needed to be removed, it felt like infertility was taking one more piece of me.

I remember lying in pre-op, staring at the ceiling, wanting to be strong, but inside, I was breaking. This wasn't just another procedure; this was final. Permanent. My fallopian tubes, the very things that were supposed to help create life, were beyond saving. My thoughts spiraled—and I couldn't stop them.

The pain after surgery was comparable to the other laparoscopies I'd endured over the years, but the emotional toll was much worse. Waking up groggy, feeling the dull, aching emptiness where my tubes used to be, I tried to tell myself this was necessary, a step forward, and that I had no other choice. But it didn't feel like progress. It felt like another cruel twist in a story I never wanted to write.

And then there was my uterus. Another surgery. Another attempt to fix what was broken.

Hysteroscopic metroplasty. Two words I had never heard before but ones that would come to define another chapter of my infertility journey. My uterus wasn't shaped correctly, and there was a large septum. A *septate* and *bicornuate* uterus, they said—something I was born with, something that could make achieving or maintaining pregnancy difficult.

I thought nothing could compare to previous surgeries, but this one nearly broke me.

The recovery was brutal. My abdomen felt like it was being torn apart from the inside out. Every movement sent sharp, radiating pain through my body. I spent days in tears, hardly able to move, trying to keep the balloon catheter in place, knowing that my uterus needed time to heal properly.

But the worst part? The waiting. I was desperate to know if the surgery had worked. Was my uterus, my body, ready to proceed with IVF? I needed reassurance that this pain meant progress, that everything I had endured wasn't for nothing. But all I could do was wait. And hope.

Because that's what infertility is—a relentless cycle of waiting, loss, and hope. Of breaking and rebuilding. Of surrendering to the unknown, even when every fiber of your being is screaming for control.

Each procedure was another piece of hope...another attempt to fix what felt so painfully broken. But as the scars healed on the outside, the wounds inside me ran deeper.

With every surgery, I lost something—my tubes, my sense of control, my belief that this would ever be easy.

And then came the emotional wounds that no surgery could fix.

Recurrent implantation failure—transferring embryos that never took. Recurrent pregnancy loss—getting a glimpse of hope only to have it ripped away. Lost embryos— tiny dreams that never got their chance. Canceled cycles, weeks of medications and preparation, only to be told it was all for nothing.

Nine rounds of injections, procedures, and heartbreak. Nine times, putting my body through the unimaginable just for a chance.

I developed a severe case of ovarian hyperstimulation syndrome (OHSS), one of the worst my doctors had seen. I was hospitalized, my abdomen swelling with fluid, my body in pain I can't even put into words. I had to undergo an unmedicated drainage, a procedure that left me gasping for breath, gripping the hospital bed rails as they removed liters of fluid.

There were days I told myself I couldn't do this anymore, that my body had endured enough, and that I didn't have the strength to face another cycle, another heartbreak, another loss.

But despite everything, I kept going. Not because I felt strong; most days I felt like I was falling apart. But deep down, buried beneath the exhaustion and pain, there was still a sliver of hope. Hope was still there, even when it felt distant, fragile, or even lost.

The Heartbreak of Failing Month After Month

Infertility has a way of shifting your entire identity. With every failed test, I felt more like a stranger in my own body.

I lost count of the nights I spent staring at the ceiling, calculating dates, cycles, and medications over and over. I avoided baby showers. Friendships grew distant. And every time someone casually asked anything about having kids, I forced a smile while my heart silently shattered.

Infertility is now a big part of my story—but it wasn't always that way. There was a time when I felt like a different version of myself, a more hopeful, less anxious, optimistic version of myself. I was a person who planned out the years, spent time on hobbies, laughed more, and was clueless about how infertility can flip your world upside down.

I miss that version of myself, but infertility stole her from me.

And that's what makes infertility so complicated.

It isn't a simple diagnosis. It's deeply layered, affecting every aspect of your life.

It's living in a fog, carrying a relentless weight, trapped in a suffocating battle between hope and despair.

With infertility comes grief for the person you once were, pain for what you're now enduring, and sadness for the path you must take. *It steals so much*. It is, in every sense, the thief of joy.

Infertility breaks you down piece by piece, forcing you to question everything: your body, your future, your identity. It strips you of control and leaves you feeling powerless, navigating a medical system that often fails to acknowledge the deep emotional wounds this journey inflicts.

Infertility isn't just a diagnosis. It's more than struggling to conceive. It's an exhausting cycle of hope and heartbreak.

Every month, you let yourself believe that maybe this time will be different. Maybe it will finally happen. And then another negative test. With each setback, the light within you dims a little more and the relentless voice inside whispers, *Will it ever be my turn?*

Dealing With the Unexpected

Infertility is an emotional, physical, and mental battle that tests your limits and forces you to carry grief few can understand.

It's watching friends move forward with their lives while you feel stuck in a painful season of waiting and disappointment. It's the quiet grief of milestones that pass you by. The loneliness of feeling like no one truly understands. And the countless sacrifices most people never have to make—just for a *chance*.

Infertility consumed every part of me. It stole my ability to be fully present, took moments I'll never get back, and left scars no one could see.

I grieved not just the years lost to infertility but the simple joys I was never given, the surprise, the ease, the ability to experience this like everyone else.

I used to imagine how I'd tell my husband I was pregnant. I pictured an exciting surprise, an intimate moment just for us, maybe a tiny onesie, a heartfelt note, or just the look in my eyes telling him everything he needed to know.

Instead, we found ourselves in doctors' offices, signing paperwork and undergoing endless tests, procedures, and treatments. There was no surprise, no spontaneous joy, just a calendar filled with appointments and a process that stripped away the magic of what we had once dreamed.

I don't remember every injection, but I remember every single way infertility made me feel. Feelings that stayed with me, shaping who I was becoming.

It made me blame myself and feel broken. It changed me in ways I never could have expected.

When Hope Feels Lost

I used to define myself by what my body couldn't do, by the ways I thought I had failed. But now, I see myself through a different lens. I am still healing, still piecing together the parts of me that infertility shattered, but I can also see the strength that carried me through.

I am someone who has endured the unimaginable and survived pain I never thought I could bear.

Infertility showed me the depths of my strength, the importance of community, and the power of advocating for myself. And while this journey will always be a part of me, it does not define me.

And it does not define you.

Infertility will test you in ways you never imagined. It will break you, reshape you, and force you to find strength in a place you didn't know existed. But if there's one thing I've learned, it's that even in the darkest moments, we keep going. Even when we don't feel strong, we fight. And that, in itself, is strength.

If you're in this place right now, know this: your pain is real, your feelings are valid, and you are not alone.

This journey may have changed me, but it didn't take me. I am still here. I am still standing. And so are you. If all you've done today is survive, that is enough too.

Chapter Two

The Infertility Rollercoaster

P eople don't realize how terrifying infertility feels. Imagine planning out your life, dreaming about your future and what it will entail, and then, in a single moment, having those dreams vanish into thin air.

What once felt certain and promising becomes a blurry mess of unknowns and what-ifs. It's like standing on solid ground one minute and being swallowed by quicksand the next, struggling to find something— anything—to hold onto.

When you're diagnosed with infertility, an overwhelming silence fills the room. You're left trying to process words you never thought you'd hear, and you're suddenly drowning in emotions while the rest of the world keeps turning, utterly unaware that your life has changed forever.

The Fear That Never Leaves You

I never knew fear like infertility. It's fear wrapped in grief and uncertainty, tangled with sadness, anger, and confusion. It feels like someone reached inside you, tore away your dreams, and left an aching void behind. Except no one around you can see it, feel it, or truly understand it.

Infertility changes everything. You don't just lose a dream; you lose a part of yourself. It's a grief that's hard to put into words. The sheer weight of it all is crushing, and you're left feeling like a shell of the person you once were, trying to navigate a life that no longer fits the picture you had painted so carefully.

You don't walk through infertility and remain the same. This entire process is a relentless emotional and mental rollercoaster. Every cycle brings a new wave of hope and fear. It feels as though you are constantly putting your life on hold yet trying not to let it take over your existence. Each milestone feels so far away, and when you get to one, it can feel hard to celebrate because this journey has stripped you of so much joy.

The Agony of Waiting

The two-week wait, that stretch of time between trying and finding out if it worked, is an excruciating state of suspense. It's a constant battle to hold onto hope while protecting yourself from disappointment.

You analyze every symptom, every twinge in your body, desperate to find some clue that this time will be different, and no matter what you tell yourself about avoiding the endless cycle of Googling, you still find yourself seeking answers that simply don't exist.

There is also pure exhaustion from medications during the treatment process. The countless injections, early morning clinic visits, alarms going off at all hours, strict protocols to follow, medication prep as if you've had injection training, and anxiety that creeps in with each pending shot—all with no guarantee.

Medications can cause bloating, weight gain, headaches, mood swings, nausea, insomnia, bruising, and countless other side effects. It is impossible to feel like yourself and even harder to process the emotions and side effects as they happen in real time.

It becomes draining not trusting your body and so frustrating waiting for your body to cooperate during the process. Then, when you suddenly stop medications, there is often a big crash that wreaks havoc on your body and mind. No one talks about the crash: it can be a confusing time with limited support.

The Sacrifices No One Sees

Infertility is heartbreaking in ways most people can't comprehend. It's conversations most people will never have to have, financial stress, major sacrifices, trying to juggle work, treatments, relationships, and more.

It's planning for futures that may never come to pass, questioning every decision you've ever made, and wondering if this is some sort of punishment for something you did wrong. It's going through grueling medical treatments only to be met with crushing heartbreak; so much feels entirely out of your control.

I remember feeling embarrassed and ashamed of my diagnosis. I didn't want to tell anyone about my infertility, afraid of judgment, awkward silences, and intrusive questions like, *Whose fault is it?* It felt like my body was failing me, as if I was broken in some fundamental way.

The shame was suffocating, and for so long, I felt utterly alone.

But here's the thing: Infertility doesn't discriminate. It doesn't care how *healthy* you are, how much you've sacrificed, or how desperately you want to be a parent. It's a cruel thief that steals your dreams and leaves you with nothing but heartache and grief. You can do everything *right* and still be handed this devastating diagnosis.

Infertility is grief. The loss of dreams. The loss of hope. The loss of the person you thought you would be. It's endless self-blame. It's feeling like your body has betrayed you in the worst possible way. It's anxiety, depression, and sleepless nights, wondering where it all went wrong. It's mental and emotional exhaustion that leaves you feeling like you're walking through life in a fog.

It's psychologically imagining two futures and trying to prepare for both outcomes.

Living in the Unknown

The emotional impact of an infertility diagnosis runs deep. There's the initial shock and disbelief that this is your reality. Then comes the grief, not just for the family you imagined, but for the life you thought you'd live.

There's anger and frustration, too: anger at your body, at the universe, at anyone who seems to get pregnant effortlessly. It can feel impossible to feel happy for others, which adds to the shame. And underneath it all is a deep, aching sense of inadequacy, a feeling that you're somehow not enough.

Coping with the uncertainty of infertility is one of the most challenging aspects of this journey. You're constantly living in limbo, not knowing what the future holds. Every decision feels monumental, and the stakes are always high. What you thought would be a sprint turns into a marathon, where you're racing against time. And everything takes *so much time.*

There's also no guarantee that even the most aggressive treatments will work, and that's a terrifying reality to live with. No one prepares you for this—or for the lack of validation you face at every stage of this journey.

You grieve, you hope, you fall apart, and you pick up the pieces again and again.

The Importance of Support

Infertility can take a toll on every aspect of your life, from your relationships to your mental health to your sense of self. It's a rollercoaster filled with incredible highs and devastating lows, testing you in ways you never imagined.

But you are not alone. There is hope, even in the darkest moments. And there is always support, even when it feels like the world doesn't understand.

Having support helped me in ways I never even knew I needed. It made all the difference during a dark time. Whether it was my partner or others who were on a similar journey, knowing I wasn't alone helped me find validation, connection, and strength. It's crucial to find people who can support you, who can offer a shoulder to cry on, or who will simply listen without judgment.

Speaking to a therapist who specializes in fertility issues can be incredibly helpful too. They can provide coping strategies, help you navigate the complex emotions that come with infertility, and offer a safe space to express your fears and frustrations. Support is an essential part that is lacking for most on this journey, but it's an aspect that can provide much-needed light.

It's also important to acknowledge that there is no right or wrong way to feel or cope with infertility and any of the thoughts, emotions, or challenges it presents. This journey is deeply personal, and whatever you're feeling is valid.

Some days, you'll feel strong and hopeful, and other days, you'll feel like you're falling apart. That's okay. Allow yourself to feel whatever you're feeling without judgment. It's okay to *not always be okay.* This path is incredibly tough, and you're doing the best you can.

And if you know someone who is dealing with infertility, be there for them. You don't have to have the right words, offer advice, or understand precisely what they're going through. Just listen. Sometimes, just knowing someone cares and is there for you is enough.

Together, we can break the silence and end the stigma surrounding infertility. We can create a world where people feel safe to share their stories and don't have to suffer in silence. We can offer each other the love, support, and understanding that is so desperately needed. No one should ever have to face this journey alone.

Chapter Three

Why Didn't Anyone Tell Me

W hen I began my fertility journey, I was naive. Un-prepared. Hopeful. Trusting. I had no idea how deeply it would affect me and test me. I underestimated the timelines, the financial strains, and the emotional toll.

For most of my life, I assumed pregnancy would be easy, and I never imagined how much IVF would test me. When it came to fertility treatments, doctors provided clinical information—a stack of paperwork, a quick consultation outlining my medication schedule, and then I was on my own. The support ended there.

Looking back, I wish someone had been honest with me from the beginning. I wish someone had prepared me rather than letting me believe any of this would be simple. Instead, I stumbled through uncertainty and the many challenges, setbacks, and losses that came my way.

Why didn't anyone prepare me for how hard this would be?

Why didn't anyone tell me that IVF isn't a guarantee? That every embryo doesn't equal a baby? That failed cycles and loss bring a heartbreak deeper than I ever imagined?

Why didn't anyone tell me how infertility seeps into every part of your life? How the emotional toll is impossible to grasp until you're in it? How the waiting feels endless, and weeks stretch into months, sometimes years? Or how infertility never fully leaves you?

These realizations blindsided me, surfacing when I least expected them. But through the devastation, they also taught me. They forced me to grow, adapt, and find strength in ways I never imagined. I wish I had known these truths earlier, but I share them with you now, so you don't have to feel as lost and alone in this as I once did.

As I reflect on my journey, there are so many lessons I wish I had learned sooner. These lessons would have shown me the power of using my voice, prioritizing my needs, and focusing on what I could control in a process that often felt so out of my hands.

Educate Yourself

There was a time when I had no idea what to expect—but I quickly realized how overwhelming this path can be. I wasn't part of support groups. I didn't have people in my life who understood what I was going through, and I wasn't aware of resources to learn more about different conditions or treatment options. But in all fairness, when I first went through infertility, there weren't online communities, podcasts, blogs, experts, or books to help explain things either.

Through personally experiencing infertility, medicated cycles, and multiple IVF cycles, I learned a lot.

But I wish I had known so much earlier on.

It felt like I was going into each test, step, and process blindly and unsure of what to expect. I believe it would have made me feel more confident, prepared, and realistic about my expectations had I known more sooner. It would have also helped me advocate for the care I deserved, the care that was often lacking. Too many times, I became trusting and compliant out of sheer ignorance rather than using my voice. Now, I encourage everyone to learn as much as they can.

It's essential to do your own research and prepare for consultations, appointments, and procedures so you feel more in control. Take the time to familiarize yourself with commonly used fertility terms, as this can make the process feel less intimidating when you're navigating treatments or connecting with others online. There are also a lot of incredible resources available now too; *use them*. Remember, an educated patient is an empowered patient.

Be Your Own Advocate

Infertility is overwhelming and confusing. When I started my fertility journey, I didn't have the confidence to speak up at the doctor's office. I hate to admit it, but there were times I didn't ask specific questions or voice concerns because I was worried about embarrassment, judgment, or treatment cycles being delayed.

But as time passed and my case became more complicated, I grew confident about speaking up.

I suddenly found myself facing recurrent implantation failure followed by recurrent pregnancy loss and realized I had no choice but to start demanding clarity and answers. I couldn't keep following the same cycle of hope and heartbreak, wishing for a different outcome. Something had to change. I knew I needed to start asking questions, demanding answers, and pushing when things didn't feel right—not just for my sanity, but *because I had every right to have a voice in my care.*

I found it helpful to compile a list of questions for appointments ahead of time, which ensured all of my questions were asked and never forgotten. Bringing a support person along to appointments was invaluable too.

I know advocating for yourself can be exhausting and even difficult at times, but it's important to remind yourself that you are putting so much on the line for this chance. You are the one taking medications, undergoing tests and procedures, and making sacrifices for this chance. Do not hesitate to advocate for yourself. *This is your journey.*

Stay Organized

Organization is crucial. It can feel like there's a lot on the go all at once because, well, *there is.* You are juggling your daily responsibilities and managing multiple medications, appointments, tests, and procedures; staying organized can significantly reduce stress and overwhelm. A few things I found helpful were having medications organized and a dedicated injection station set up at home. This simplified the medication aspect for me.

Having a calendar highlighting my protocol, medications, and important dates helped me plan for the days and months ahead.

Finally, keeping detailed notes on appointments, medication schedules, hormone levels, ultrasound results, egg retrieval results, embryology outcomes, and expected procedure dates was also incredibly beneficial. These steps allowed me to feel organized and prepared, especially when navigating multiple rounds of IVF.

Don't Stop Living

Infertility is one chapter, not your whole story.

There was a point during my darkest season when I realized that I had stopped living. I was in survival mode, racing against time, going through the motions month after month, no longer doing anything I once loved. I was lost and broken.

I began to reflect on the years that had passed, the experiences I wasn't present for because I was entirely consumed by infertility, and the irretrievable moments I had missed out on. There is grief in this moment. A pain that adds to the weight we already carry.

I wish I had understood sooner that infertility is a marathon, not a sprint. It was unwise putting my whole life on pause, waiting for an outcome I couldn't control. If you feel it's too late, that you have already stopped living, know that you can start now. You will never be able to reclaim time, but learning to live and find joy now, despite the heaviness and uncertainty, is crucial.

Start by setting small, non-fertility-related goals like picking up a hobby you've put off or even something as simple as scheduling a coffee date with a friend. Look for moments that bring joy and remember to celebrate along the way too. Whether it's taking your first shot, embryo transfer day, or small wins outside of infertility, don't stop living and celebrating what's happening *now*.

Don't Compare Your Journey

I know it's hard not to compare yourself to others; I've been there countless times too.

At one point, I compared *everything*: how easily others got pregnant, what supplements others took during successful cycles—even bizarre rituals people swore by. Desperation made me cling to the idea that *if it worked for them, maybe it would work for me.* It's easy to get caught up and carried away with comparisons, especially within the scope of social media.

Comparison is hard. I get it. But it's important to remind yourself that no two journeys are the same. Everyone's path is different and unique, including yours. Comparison isn't helpful; it can add layers of stress, envy, sadness, jealousy, and frustration. *Do not allow it to consume you.*

Prioritize Your Mental Health

I'm fine. I'm good. I'm okay. How many times have you said these words while fighting back tears? How many times have you forced a smile while feeling like your world is collapsing, struggling to catch your breath? How many times have you said those words after another negative pregnancy test, another obstacle, or another piece of heartbreaking news?

Infertility is often years of disappointment, pain, fear, emptiness, and grief, which does not equal being *okay*. It's traumatic and a daily battle, which can leave you feeling paralyzed. You'll have good days, bad days, and can't-get-out-of-bed days. Struggling doesn't mean you're failing.

For so long, I pretended to be okay. Smiling on the outside while struggling on the inside. Silently carrying the weight of it all. But one day, I realized that pretending wasn't helping anyone, especially me. I recognized the importance of taking steps to prioritize and protect my mental health.

I learned to say *no* to situations that drained me. I gave myself permission to take breaks, whether that meant skipping a baby shower or stepping away from social media. I started setting aside time for myself, like daily walks, journaling my thoughts, and utilizing support that allowed me to process the grief.

And I made a point to practice daily affirmations and positive self-talk. Despite feeling forced, they served as important reminders. I encourage you to try these too: *My feelings are valid. I am doing my best, and that is enough. I am not alone in this. I am more than my struggle. I am loved. I am worthy of joy.*

Find Support

Infertility is a rollercoaster. The ups, downs, waiting, hopes, and heartbreaks can be excruciating. Many of us didn't realize how much we need support until we found it.

Infertility can make you feel like you have to do this alone, but you don't. The right people can make all the difference. Surround yourself with those who lift you up, and lean into those who truly understand. Support looks different for everyone, and there is no one-size-fits-all approach. What matters most is recognizing what you need and honoring that. Trust your instincts, ask questions, and push for the care and validation you deserve.

As hard as it is, celebrate your small wins, grieve every loss, and allow yourself to feel everything this journey brings. Infertility trauma runs deep. It's often years of pain, doubt, fear, living in survival mode, and struggling with continuous hardships. Be kind to yourself. Give yourself the same love and compassion you would give to someone else in your shoes.

If you are in this right now, I hope these lessons bring you even the smallest glimmer of light. They won't erase the pain, but they may help you stand a little taller, breathe a little deeper, and face another day.

Infertility will test you in ways you never imagined, but remember: It does not define you. There is strength in knowledge, power in advocating for yourself, and healing in allowing yourself to be supported.

Chapter Four

Fertility Confessions

F or so much of my infertility journey, I felt utterly alone—not just in the experience itself but in the thoughts I kept buried, the emotions I couldn't explain, and the truths I didn't dare say out loud.

The world around me felt different, as if I'd been dropped into an alternate reality, one that no one else could see or understand. I was surrounded by people yet completely isolated, carrying a grief so heavy that words couldn't express.

But the hardest part wasn't just the sadness; it was the silence. No one talks about this. No one tells you how infertility changes you, turning the simplest moments into triggers or the way it makes you feel like a stranger in your own body. How it forces you to carry pain so deep yet so invisible.

This chapter isn't just about infertility. It's about the things we *don't say*, the things so many of us feel but are too afraid to admit because we feel alone.

The Things We Don't Say

When infertility first entered my life, I tried to convince myself that I could still be the same person. I could show up to social events, smile, and pretend like nothing had changed. But infertility has a way of seeping into every part of you, reshaping how you experience the world.

I used to love catching up with friends, but infertility changed that. It made me feel boring, a person others avoided because my presence carried a heaviness no one could sit with. Conversations that once felt effortless now left me feeling like an outsider. Every discussion seemed to circle back to milestones I couldn't reach: pregnancy symptoms, baby names, sleepless nights with a newborn.

But it wasn't just the talk of babies. It was everything. Taking trips, buying homes, big promotions. Milestone after milestone. Life kept moving forward for everyone except me.

I wasn't just missing out on motherhood; I was losing the ability to connect with the people in my life. Every outing, every gathering, every holiday became another heavy reminder of that.

I felt disconnected, out of sync in conversations, and unable to relate. The excitement I once had for life felt distant, replaced by a quiet sadness that seemed to follow me everywhere.

And here's the part I never admitted for so long: I never thought I would feel jealous of my best friend. I never thought I would feel sick to my stomach seeing a pregnancy announcement. I never thought I would have to fake a smile while celebrating a family member, only to go home and cry.

But I did. And for the longest time, I thought that made me a bad person.

Infertility makes you feel like you are drowning in a sea of emotions you don't recognize. Resentment. Bitterness. Anger. The kind of feelings you don't want to admit because they make you feel small, ashamed, ungrateful.

But here's the truth: You can be happy for someone else and heartbroken for yourself at the same time. You can love your pregnant friend and still cry after seeing her ultrasound photo. You can attend a baby shower and still feel like you can't breathe. You can feel joy for others and grief for yourself, and neither cancels the other out.

Exhausting Encounters

Infertility tested every relationship in my life.

My marriage, once filled with lighthearted conversations about the future, became consumed with medical appointments, financial stress, and heartbreak.

Friends drifted away, not knowing how to support me. Others tried to be helpful but often said the wrong things. Even my family, though well-meaning, didn't understand the emotional toll in any capacity.

I continuously fought to keep everything inside yet wanted nothing more than to cry and say out loud just how hard this was.

People kept telling me, *You're so strong.* But I didn't feel strong; I was just surviving. And some days, even that felt like too much.

Socializing became overwhelming, and being around people was draining. I was exhausted from pretending to be okay, forcing a smile while breaking inside. I was tired of hearing unhelpful advice that made it seem like a simple solution existed for something so excruciating or being told that *everything would be fine* when no one could possibly know that.

So I pulled away. It was easier to hide away than to pretend.

Infertility Made Me Someone I Didn't Recognize

I used to be lighthearted, optimistic, the glass-half-full person always believing things would work out. Infertility stole that from me. I became angry in ways I never had before.

I resented strangers. I avoided social events because I couldn't bear another conversation about pregnancy, kids, or family life. I felt like a shell of the person I used to be.

I was bitter. I was exhausted. And worst of all, I felt like I was failing, not just at getting pregnant, but at holding onto the person I once was.

Infertility steals so much: time, money, relationships, joy, and pieces of yourself you never imagined losing. It occupied my mind, filling every quiet moment with doubt and longing.

Every day, I felt at war with myself. Dark thoughts were constant, each one pulling me deeper into anxiety, isolation, and self-blame. *What did I do to deserve this? Why am I being punished? Why her and not me? My husband would be better off without me. Will I ever feel true happiness again? This is my fault.*

It made me feel like I was losing myself. I used to find joy in the little things. Curling up with a book, baking a new recipe, attending local events, decorating for the holidays. But as infertility consumed more of my mind, those things slipped away too.

I stopped reading because I couldn't focus. I stopped traveling because every dollar went toward treatments. I stopped making plans for the future because I no longer knew what the future held. I stopped buying new clothes because I kept telling myself that *maybe next year I'll be pregnant.*

My life became measured in treatment cycles, testing days, and endless *what-ifs*, each one dictating my next move. While everyone else seemed to move forward, I was stuck, holding my breath, waiting.

I don't think people understand how terrifying and heartbreaking it is to live this way. It makes you continuously feel behind in life, and the sacrifices you make along the way (that no one seems to see or understand) amplify this feeling.

I remember one day standing in front of the mirror, staring at my reflection and thinking, *Who am I?* It felt like I was disappearing, piece by piece, replaced by someone I no longer recognized.

And I kept all of it inside.

Pretending to Be Okay

I was constantly overwhelmed by thoughts and emotions I couldn't control.

There were countless times I hid away crying in the bathroom, eyes red and puffy, thoughts filled with pain and heartbreak. Then I'd collect myself, wipe away the tears, take a deep breath, and step back out into the world like nothing was wrong.

There were so many times I wanted to scream. *Does anyone see how hard this is? I'm exhausted from fighting every single day for something that comes so easily to everyone else.*

I wanted to admit that some days, I was so tired of hoping, and I didn't know if I had the strength to keep going.

But I never said those things because infertility teaches you to stay quiet, to pretend, to hold it all in. The world isn't built to embrace this kind of pain.

You can receive the most devastating news of your life and still be expected to move forward as if nothing has happened—because no one seems to acknowledge or understand the pain this journey brings.

Infertility is waking up every day wondering, *When will it be my turn?* And sleepless nights questioning, *What if it never is?*

It's feeling like a stranger in your own life because nothing feels the way it used to.

Faking a smile at a baby shower while your heart shatters inside.

Feeling guilty for the way infertility has changed you, even though it's not your fault.

Carrying a pain so deep, yet so invisible, that most people will never know you are falling apart right in front of them.

The Triggers No One Warns You About

Infertility has a way of making everything more painful. I felt an intense sadness and anger I never knew existed, and at the same time, everything around me became more excruciating.

Triggers hit at any moment. Scrolling on social media and seeing a pregnancy announcement, walking past the baby aisle while shopping, seeing a baby commercial on TV, or just overhearing a stranger talking about morning sickness.

Then there were birthdays. I began to hate my birthday. Each passing year became another reminder that my one wish still hadn't come true. Every year that passed felt heavier. I used to love celebrating birthdays, but now they just marked another year of waiting.

These weren't just reminders of what I didn't have. Each felt like a loss I had to grieve over and over again.

I learned to master the art of holding it together in public, only to collapse into tears as soon as I got home.

Infertility already feels like the most unfair thing imaginable. Add in holidays, baby announcements, or celebratory days, and life can become impossible.

People say, *sad for me, happy for you,* but sometimes it's just *sad for me,* **not** *happy for you.* And that's a truth many of us live with, even if no one talks about it.

Infertility comes with grief that never fully leaves you, but it also comes with guilt.

Guilt for the way you feel, for the friendships you let fade because you couldn't handle another pregnancy update. Guilt for the resentment you carry, even when you don't want to. Guilt for the way infertility affects your marriage, your happiness, and your ability to be present. Guilt for the parts of yourself you've lost along the way.

I have spent so many nights lying awake, wondering if I was being selfish, if I was being unfair. Wondering if maybe they were right.

Maybe I should have been stronger, more grateful. Perhaps I should have just been happy for them without the ache in my chest. Possibly, if I had handled it better, I wouldn't feel so alone.

But infertility takes pieces of you. It changes the way you love, the way you connect, the way you see the world. *And it's okay to admit that.*

The Weight of Misunderstanding

Infertility is one of the most profoundly misunderstood experiences a person can endure. It's not just the physical toll or the endless uncertainty; it's the way the world responds to it. The way people fail to understand the weight we carry.

Instead of compassion, we are met with advice we didn't ask for. Instead of understanding, we are met with dismissal. Instead of support, we are met with silence.

It is a condition that pushes so much blame onto the person suffering, as if it's something we caused, something we could fix if only we *relaxed* or *stopped stressing*. But infertility is not our fault. It is not a mindset issue or a problem that can be solved with optimism.

And yet, we are made to feel as though it is.

We are expected to carry this pain quietly. To show up to baby showers, to celebrate milestones we are aching for, to smile and be happy for others while carrying the unbearable weight of our grief. We are expected to push aside our pain while putting everyone else's joy above our heartbreak.

Infertility pushes you beyond limits you never imagined you had. It forces you to keep going when you have nothing left to give, isolating you in ways that no one talks about. And in the moments when you need support the most, it can feel like the world has turned away, leaving you to carry it all alone.

But you are not alone. And this is not your fault.

Finding Strength in the Hardest Moments

This journey is unfair. It's exhausting. It's heartbreaking in ways most people will never understand. Infertility changes you, breaking you down, reshaping your identity, and forcing you to confront grief that few acknowledge. You grieve the life you thought you'd have, the person you used to be, the experiences you imagined so clearly but might never get.

And the hardest part? Most people don't see it as grief at all.

So they say nothing. They don't bring comfort; they don't check in or acknowledge the loss. And you're left carrying this invisible grief alone, pretending you're okay when you're *anything but* okay. But let me remind you: this grief is real, and your pain is real.

But grief isn't the whole story.

Infertility tried to break me, but it also built me in ways I never expected. It forced me to advocate for myself, to set boundaries, to choose carefully who I allowed into my most vulnerable moments. Some days, strength looked like showing up to an appointment. Other days, it was simply getting out of bed.

And then there were moments, small ones, where I felt hope. A kind word from a stranger. A nurse who took an extra moment to comfort me. A conversation where someone didn't try to fix it but simply sat with me in the pain. A quiet walk where, for just a moment, I could breathe.

Hope wasn't loud or obvious. It was quiet, sometimes barely noticeable. But it was there.

If you've ever felt these things, if you've carried these thoughts in silence, if you've ever wondered if you were the only one experiencing these emotions, you are not alone.

You are allowed to feel every single emotion without guilt, without shame, without apology.

My hope is that these words have given you even the smallest piece of validation. You are not broken. You are never alone. Even in the hardest moments, there are others right there with you.

And if you need to step away, cry, breathe, or collect yourself, know that it's okay. You are carrying a weight unlike any other. I have been there, too, and one day, this heaviness won't define you. One day, you'll step back out, and while the weight may never fully disappear, it won't consume you anymore.

No matter where you are on this journey, you are never alone in it. I know, because I've been there too.

Chapter Five

The Waiting Game

N othing could have prepared me for the agonizing wait.

Infertility is an inescapable cycle of waiting. Waiting to conceive, waiting for results, waiting for answers. I lost count of how many two-week-waits I endured over the years. From the hopeful early days of trying to the many IVF embryo transfers, each one held the same breath-stealing anticipation. And then there were the in-betweens. The moments where time seemed to stand still, suspended between hope and heartbreak.

Despite the countless waiting periods over the years, I still remember my first big wait. Month one of a medicated at-home cycle. At the time, I had to advocate just to try medication, given my *age* and *health*, so it felt like a major milestone. A moment filled with hope.

Yes, I needed help to get pregnant, but it didn't feel like the end of the world. We could still try at home, and surely, it would happen, right? Whether it was the doctors reassuring me or my own ignorance about the real odds of conceiving each month, I *truly* believed this would be the cycle.

So many plans and dreams had formed in my mind already. Little did I know that this wouldn't be the cycle to bring us any closer to pregnancy, and neither would the months to follow. This was the beginning of a much longer journey. A journey filled with endless waiting.

Endless Waiting

As time passed, anxiety took hold, accompanied by fear and worry. Each month felt endless, and every negative test pushed my dreams further out of reach. It was around this time that infertility started affecting me in ways I never could have imagined.

With each passing month, my mindset shifted, my relationships became more strained, and the dread of another negative test consumed my thoughts. Then came the grief of yet another period. I had never heard this grief talked about; before then, I hadn't known it existed.

I began to have complicated feelings about pregnancy announcements. I started to wonder why others could get pregnant but not me. Fear, worry, hope, and sadness intertwined, consuming me. It felt devastating.

Eventually, waiting took on a whole new meaning. Navigating fertility treatment cycles came with even higher stakes financially, mentally, and emotionally. The mix of emotions from the early days became amplified beyond anything I had ever anticipated.

My calendars were packed with treatment protocols and medication schedules. My phone constantly buzzed with reminders. My days were filled with appointments and procedures. And despite the nonstop cycle of it all, I was always waiting. Waiting for the next step, the next call, the next chance.

What I didn't expect was the sheer amount of waiting both before a cycle and during one—waiting for my period to start, waiting for next steps, waiting for medications to begin. There was waiting for embryology updates or lab results. It was *endless*.

It was impossible to plan anything around it. My life revolved around waiting, yet I wasn't sure how to process the emotions. I just kept moving forward, hoping we were finally on the right path.

The Emotional Toll of the Two-Week Wait

Then came the two-week-waits during fertility treatments, when time seemed to stop.. As patients, we follow such strict schedules, time-sensitive medications, meticulously planned procedures, everything structured to the smallest detail. But after embryo transfer day, there was nothing.

For two full weeks, there were no more appointments or tests, just time standing still, thick with unknowns and uncertainty. With everything on the line and so much invested in this one chance, the wait became an emotional rollercoaster, an impossibly trying cycle of what-ifs and maybes as testing day loomed.

It was a delicate balancing act. I teetered between staying busy to distract myself, taking it day by day, adjusting my lifestyle as if I was already pregnant, battling intrusive thoughts and anxiety, overanalyzing every sensation, and trying my hardest to avoid Google. Each moment was a fragile line between holding onto hope and bracing for disappointment, all while navigating some of the heaviest emotions I had ever faced.

Finding Ways to Cope

I learned that the emotional toll of infertility and the two-week wait can be overwhelming, making it easy to lose sight of your own well-being. But prioritizing yourself, even in small ways, is essential.

Finding moments of calm, setting boundaries, and focusing on what you can control can make a difference in navigating this difficult wait.

It's easy to get sucked into symptom-spotting and endless online searches. However, it's so beneficial to resist the urge to turn to Google or online forums for every symptom, question, or concern. The internet can quickly become a rabbit hole of conflicting information, and what starts as a simple search can lead to heightened emotions. Instead of helping, it often adds confusion to an already emotional process.

It's natural to seek reassurance by looking at other people's experiences, but comparisons rarely bring peace. No two journeys are the same, and symptom-spotting based on someone else's experience can add unnecessary stress and disappointment. Finding healthy distractions can help.

It's about finding moments of peace and joy in the wait, even if only for a little while.

Remember, everyone's body and journey are different. Comparing your symptoms and timeline to someone else's only adds unnecessary stress and disappointment. Try to limit your time online and be mindful that it might be adding more to your mental load.

Self-care isn't just spa days; it's about protecting your mental health and allowing yourself moments of peace, especially during difficult seasons. Whether that's by enjoying a quiet walk, journaling, reading, or stepping away from social media, self-care is vital. Infertility takes so much, but caring for yourself is one thing you can control. Give yourself permission to rest and reset. You are worthy of this time and care.

Acknowledge that the two-week-wait is incredibly stressful, and it's completely normal to feel a range of emotions from sadness to hope. Allow yourself to experience these emotions fully, without judgment. It's important to understand that no emotion is wrong or invalid. You may feel hope one moment and doubt the next, and that's okay.

Sometimes, the emotional highs and lows can feel like they're too much to carry, but remember it's okay to take a break from them too. You don't have to feel everything all the time. It's about finding balance, knowing when to lean into those emotions and when to give yourself a little room to breathe. Remind yourself that you're doing the best you can.

Facing Testing Day

There's also the question of testing. For me, I had to know. It gave me a sense of control in an uncontrollable process. I needed to prepare my mind and heart before the clinic knew too. But testing also brought more anxiety, stress, and worry. It was easy to obsess over these results and feel the need to retest too.

Deciding whether or not to test at home is deeply personal. Some prefer to wait for the fertility clinic's blood work results, while others choose to test early to prepare themselves for the outcome. Some arrange for a voice message to be left, so they can hear the news when they feel ready, while others rely on a partner to take the call. There's no right or wrong way, only what feels best for you.

When it comes to pregnancy testing day (or BETA Day), it can be helpful to prepare emotionally for any outcome. Whether the result is positive or negative, it can be an intensely charged moment. So much blood, so many tears, and so many sacrifices have gone into this moment.

Managing expectations during this wait and testing period is critical. If your results are positive, allow yourself to feel joy and excitement, but also acknowledge that it's natural to have mixed emotions. A positive test doesn't erase the pain of this journey or make everything suddenly simple or okay.

If your results are negative, it's important to give yourself permission to grieve and feel it all. The heartbreak from a failed cycle is devastating. It is a profound loss that many don't understand, but know that your pain is real and what you're feeling is valid. Take time to process your emotions.

Infertility is waiting. Waiting for answers, waiting for results, waiting for a dream that feels *just* out of reach. It's exhausting, unpredictable, and deeply unfair. And some days, the waiting will feel impossible. But even in the hardest moments, remember that you are doing the best you can. One step at a time, one breath at a time—keep moving forward, knowing that you are never alone.

Chapter Six

When Infertility Tests Everything

I've struggled to put into words everything I have to say about relationships and infertility. I've rewritten this chapter numerous times, trying to piece the words together to make perfect sense. Then my thoughts scatter, and my emotions become conflicted as I reflect on the disruption, heartache, and loss infertility has caused here.

There is so much to say, so many layers, and a profound ripple effect that impacts the relationships around you when you go through infertility. I've realized that just like the words written in this chapter, real-life relationships are complex, and making sense of it all within a single chapter feels impossible, but I'll try.

Infertility and the Battle Within

Infertility seeps into every aspect of your existence. It's the constant ache deep within your heart, wondering if it will ever be your turn. The constant cycle of hope and heartbreak. The silent grief during holidays, baby showers, and anytime you hear a pregnancy announcement.

The sadness and frustration that lingers with every well-meaning but unhelpful piece of advice, and the anxiety that never fully fades. The invisible weight of infertility can consume every conversation, interaction, and thought. It completely reshapes how you see yourself, your relationships, and the world around you.

It's easy to spiral into self-blame, questioning your worth and feeling like your body has betrayed you. Even when you know, deep down, it's not your fault, it can still feel like it is. Thoughts like *My partner would be better off without me, Maybe I'm not meant to be a mom,* and *What did I do to deserve this?* take over. And in the darkest moments, blame can feel justified, offering a false sense of control in an uncontrollable process.

Infertility amplifies every emotion—anger, resentment, comparison, hope, and fear.

Fear of being *that* couple who never had kids. Fear of being left behind. Fear that you're failing your partner. Fear that you'll never find joy again. Anger that people oversimplify it. Anger that your emotions are dismissed and your pain minimized. Anger at how easy it seems for others, at your body for not cooperating, and at the sacrifices that never seem to end. Then there's rage, the kind that comes from having no control over your life.

This process can quickly make you into an angry, bitter person because it feels like you are fighting for your life every single day.

This journey is brutal, mentally exhausting, and isolating in ways you never imagined. Infertility makes you feel like you don't fit in. Resentment creeps in toward friends who don't understand, partners who don't physically endure it, and the overwhelming unfairness of it all.

Comparison becomes inevitable. Each pregnancy announcement or social media post can feel like salt in an open wound. It's hard not to wonder, *Why them and not me?* It's normal to feel grief, sadness, and guilt when you see others' joy, even while struggling with your own pain. But it's important to remember that these emotions are not mutually exclusive; they coexist. They don't make you a bad person. They make you human.

Grief, Isolation, and Misunderstanding

Infertility is often fought silently, but wow, is it ever loud. It consumes you in ways you could never imagine. You quite often feel at war with yourself. Over time, sadness, despair, and uncertainty take hold, and you grieve for the person you once were.

But instead of receiving support for this profound loss, we are often met with opinions, stigma, and blame. Even those closest to us may minimize our pain, offer simplistic advice, or invalidate our experiences with toxic positivity. *Just relax. Have you tried...? Everything happens for a reason. You can always adopt.* These comments become so normalized and frequent that, over time, they can spark frustration and even anger. How could anyone not have difficult thoughts and emotions in response?

All we really need is a simple *I'm sorry, I'm here for you* or someone to listen without trying to fix the problem. But because infertility is so misunderstood and its effects underestimated, many of us are left to grieve silently.

Even thinking about being surrounded by people and their comments and questions can be anxiety-inducing. You may even start avoiding gatherings altogether because it's easier to isolate and protect your heart.

Then with each passing month, you watch those around you continue to move forward as you watch yourself slip further away.

Infertility grief flows into every relationship. There is grief over lost friendships. There is grief over the absence of support from those you expected to be there for you when you needed them the most. Friends who once felt like lifelines may seem distant, not because they don't care but because they don't know how to show up for you anymore. It's an unintentional abandonment, and it stings.

Sharing Your Story on Your Terms

For some, sharing what they're experiencing can bring relief and connection. For others, it brings pressure and fear of judgment. This decision is deeply personal and unique, which is why deciding what feels right for you is important.

The first and most important thing to know here is that sharing your story is never a requirement. It's a personal choice and should be a decision you make for yourself. I'm often asked about sharing my story with friends or family. *Was it easy? How much did you share? What if someone expects updates, and you're not ready? Did you ever regret telling someone?*

Sharing our struggles with others can come with a lot of thoughts and emotions. Just like experiencing infertility, sharing can feel full of unknowns and uncertainty. It can also feel scary to say certain things out loud. For me, saying what I was going through to others initially made everything feel that much more real. There were a lot of tears and big emotions telling people, but a weight was also lifted.

As time went on and treatments began, there were cycles where I felt lighter sharing and others when keeping things private was the only way to cope because I was not ready to share the weight of another devastating setback, loss, or harsh reality. In time, I realized that both of these are okay and necessary.

There may always be people in your life who simply never understand. I've encountered countless people questioning my choices, and at times, their words got in my head. I found myself second-guessing my decisions, wondering if maybe they were right.

But I've learned that it's easy for others to judge a situation they've never experienced. It's easy to say "just do this" or "why not that." I've also come to realize that it's okay if no one around you truly gets it. One day, the same people asking you *why* will be the ones asking you *how* you did it.

How others feel about it isn't your responsibility. This is your journey. The only voice that matters is your own.

Boundaries and communication become a lifeline. Just because you share what you're going through once doesn't mean others are entitled to regular updates. If someone oversteps, it's okay to speak up or walk away.

If someone pries or offers unsolicited advice, having a simple response ready can be empowering. You might say, *I'll update you when I'm ready to talk again* or *I'd rather not discuss that.* If someone makes you feel unsupported or judged, it's okay to pull back. Your boundaries are valid, and you have every right to protect your peace.

Remember, you don't owe anyone an explanation. You have the right to choose what parts of your journey you share and when to share them.

Difficult Conversations and Tough Decisions

For some couples, infertility can bring you closer together, but for many, it can pull you in separate ways.

I didn't think infertility would affect my relationship the way it did. It's not just the physical toll of fertility treatments or the monthly hope-crushing reality of another negative pregnancy test, it's the continuous cycle of uncertainty, sacrifices, and grief that you both face.

It's the heartbreak of watching your partner silently struggle, the overwhelming thoughts that you aren't enough, and the consuming reality that this might not ever happen for you.

It's the physical toll from fertility treatments, which one partner often bears more heavily. The continuous medications, tests, and probing can make love feel clinical and cold, slowly stripping away the magic of intimacy.

There's also a unique pain in feeling like you're failing the person you love. I often felt like I was the cause of our heartbreak, that if I could just fix whatever was broken in me, our life would go back to normal.

There were moments where I convinced myself that my partner would be happier without me, and countless moments where I felt less than because my body wouldn't do the one thing that came so easily for everyone else.

Infertility tests even the strongest relationships. It is one of the hardest challenges any couple can face together. It forces conversations most people never will: *How much money are we willing to spend? How many treatments do we want to try? What if none of them work? Are we going to be okay? What if one of us wants to stop trying and the other doesn't? What happens to our embryos in case of death or divorce?*

Infertility doesn't care how much you love each other, how many sacrifices you make, or how much you want a child. It's ruthless and relentless. But despite these immense challenges, learning to communicate and work together as a team is crucial. At the end of the day, that's what you are—a team, even when it's easy to lose sight of that while trying to survive.

Love, Uncertainty, and Connection

People deal with life's difficult experiences differently; it's what makes us human. Infertility is no exception. Two people in a relationship can, and often do, deal with this path in different ways. One partner may want to talk everything out, while the other shuts down. One may stay hopeful, while the other anticipates the worst.

Though it can feel scary to admit that you're struggling as a couple, know that you are not alone. Sadly, this is just another aspect of infertility that is rarely spoken about. Sometimes, love isn't about having all the answers; it's about holding each other through the uncertainty. It's important to work through this together, so you can find ways to support each other and help prevent resentment and emotional distance.

One way to reconnect is by planning regular date nights or scheduling infertility-free time. This means having moments where you don't talk about infertility, treatments, appointments, or the emotions tied to your journey. These simple moments together are a reminder of the foundation of your relationship, the connection that existed before infertility took center stage.

Another important way to stay connected is by checking in with each other. Ask your partner how they're feeling—not just about the treatments but about life in general. Make space for honest, vulnerable conversations, and let each other share emotions, even when it's hard to find the right words. Remember, opening up creates intimacy and trust, helping both of you feel heard and supported in this difficult chapter.

Communication is key for all relationships. These conversations might be tough, but they're absolutely necessary. The only way to get through this together is to talk about it. Share your struggles with your partner. Let them know when you need extra support. And make sure to ask how they're doing too. Infertility impacts you both, even if it looks different for each person.

And don't overlook the power of counseling. Couples therapy can be a safe, neutral space to work through the emotional complexities of infertility together. It allows you both to share your fears, frustrations, and hopes without judgment.

You Are Not Broken

I never expected infertility to impact my relationships, including the one with myself.

For so long, I felt broken and lost. I didn't recognize myself in the mirror. I hated my body, blamed myself, felt unfixable, and convinced myself that I would never experience happiness again. Infertility changed me to my core. It made me feel as though nothing else mattered. It stole from me, and what once brought me joy seemed insignificant compared to the all-consuming path I was currently on.

For so long, I kept silent and felt as though the thoughts, emotions, and experiences I was struggling with were unique. I felt alone with this. It added an even heavier layer to what I was already going through. With this came more shame, guilt, and isolation.

But infertility is common, and these thoughts and emotions are common, yet no one talks about it. No one talks about how infertility changes you, how it stays with you, how it impacts your relationships and the world around you. But we need to.

There are so many layers to infertility that aren't spoken about, and for far too long, we have been left to struggle silently, left to feel broken. But speaking about these devastatingly common challenges helps normalize them for others.

Infertility changed me, but I now know that infertility isn't my fault. Words I wish I'd heard and comprehended a long time ago. Words I wish everyone on this path would hear and understand.

If you're currently facing this, know that you are not broken. Struggling does not mean you are failing. This is an impossible thing to go through without feeling the weight of it all.

If you're feeling lost and as though happiness is out of reach, reconnecting with yourself is a vital step toward healing. But I won't lie; it isn't easy. When you're consumed by infertility, it can feel impossible to focus on anything else. But the truth is, infertility already takes so much—you don't have to hand over every part of yourself too.

Start by journaling about your non-fertility goals. Write down the dreams and aspirations that make you uniquely you. Maybe it's learning a new skill, joining a book club, starting a new class, or even revisiting a hobby you've always wanted to explore.

Infertility can be emotionally taxing, and it's easy to lose sight of who you are outside of this. These reflections can help you reconnect with the person you are beyond your infertility journey. You have to remind yourself that you are more than your diagnosis.

Scheduling intentional *me-time* is another simple way to emotionally check in with yourself. Set aside time each week that's entirely for you. No distractions, no expectations.

Whether it's soaking in a warm bath, mindful meditation, disconnecting from noise, hiking through nature, reading a book, or rediscovering passions that have nothing to do with your fertility journey, these moments are essential.

Having me-time allows your body and mind to slow down, so you can sit with your feelings, process emotions, and prioritize what you truly need.

And if you're reading this and feeling stuck, start small. One thing. One moment. One breath of space that is just for you. You are not lost forever. You are still here, still you, even if you feel like pieces of yourself have faded. Rebuilding takes time, but you are worth every step forward, even the smallest ones.

The impact of infertility on relationships is profound and painful, but it's also an opportunity to grow closer to those who truly support you, deepen your self-awareness, and find strength you never knew you had.

As you navigate this journey, give yourself grace. Lean into relationships that nurture you. Embrace those who offer understanding and comfort. Distance yourself from those who don't, and remember that infertility doesn't define you. You are more than your diagnosis.

As I mentioned at the beginning of this chapter, relationships are deeply complex. Capturing everything in a single chapter, finding the perfect words, and making sense of it all within these pages feels impossible—there's simply too much to say. But my hope is that in sharing my heart, you find comfort in knowing you are never alone.

Chapter Seven

The Mental Toll

Infertility stripped away everything, piece by piece, until the life I once envisioned became a distant memory.

No one prepares you for this.

For the way infertility seeps into every part of you, reshaping not only your body but also your mind, identity, and sense of self-worth. For the way it forces you into a battle you never signed up for, one that leaves scars no one else can see.

I've spent years as both a counselor and a patient, and yet, nothing could have prepared me for how deeply infertility would invade my mental and emotional well-being.

I have sat with people at their lowest moments, tears falling down their faces, their voices barely above a whisper. I have seen people who feel completely broken, numb to the world, convinced they can't make it through another day. I have witnessed pain in patients' eyes that I never thought would affect me, too, a sadness so isolating that it feels like no one else could understand.

I have seen the happiest-looking people fall apart. I have seen the most lost people find a way to build themselves back up. I have sat with the pain, heartache, and unspoken grief and carried them with me forever. It's impossible to forget these moments.

Despite knowing all of this and having years of experience working with people in their hardest moments, nothing could have prepared me for the way infertility would break me from the inside out. How it would turn me into the very person I once supported.

The one drowning in grief.

The one questioning their purpose.

The one fighting to get through another day.

Infertility isn't just about struggling to conceive. It impacts your mental health in ways few understand. Studies show that women experiencing infertility are at significantly higher risk for anxiety, depression, and psychological distress, with research comparing the emotional toll to that of individuals navigating life-threatening illnesses.

And yet, mental health is still an overlooked aspect of this experience.

When we talk about infertility, the focus is almost always on the physical effects, the medications, the procedures, the endless tests. But what about the emotional toll?

The trauma that runs deep and never fully fades.

The grief that lingers, unacknowledged.

The loneliness that isolates you, even in a crowded room.

Why is this part of the journey so rarely discussed?

The Unseen Struggle

Infertility has made me lose confidence in my body. It has made me hate my body in ways I never thought possible. During this journey, I ended up in one of the darkest mental health states I have ever experienced.

There is still so much stigma and shame surrounding infertility, and when mental health struggles are added to the mix, the loneliness only deepens.

Anxiety whispers: *What if this never happens for me?*

Depression echoes: *I don't even know who I am anymore.*

Shame convinces you: *I should be stronger than this.*

Guilt reminds you: *Maybe I should just be happy for others without the ache in my chest that won't go away.*

No one warns you that opposite emotions can coexist. That you can feel hope and fear, gratitude and anger, love and resentment all at once.

It's all I think about. I feel sad all the time, like joy is something I can no longer reach. I feel empty inside. I struggle to determine if it's anxiety or if my feelings are justified. Even positive moments in this process feel negative because I'm always stuck wondering what's next.

Infertility is a persistent battle within. There's an overwhelming mix of fear and anxiety that stems from the endless unknowns and what-ifs. You are often left alone with your thoughts, questioning everything. *Why does it come so easily for everyone else but not for me? Why am I being punished? Will this ever happen for me?*

Infertility filled me with sadness, but I carried it as anger. It was easier to be angry than to admit how deeply I was grieving. It becomes painful to watch the world move forward while you remain stuck, feeling as though life is passing you by.

I spent years pretending to be okay, pretending I wasn't breaking, holding back tears while the weight of infertility suffocated me.

I sat in countless fertility clinic waiting rooms, surrounded by other women whose eyes held the same quiet grief. We were given protocols, medications, and statistics. But no one asked how we were coping. No one prepared us for the emotional aftermath of a failed cycle, loss, or the loneliness that swallowed us whole between appointments.

When Infertility Consumes You

At one point, infertility consumed every part of me. I stopped living, stopped finding joy, and lost sight of the person I once was. It became my entire identity. It felt impossible to think about anything else. I was a stranger to myself.

Loss after loss. Failure after failure. Each negative test, each devastating phone call, and each passing month chipped away at me until I felt like there was nothing left.

At first, I didn't even notice it happening. I kept moving forward, convincing myself I was okay, that I was *strong* enough to handle it.

But infertility can break you in slow, quiet ways. It doesn't destroy you all at once. It takes pieces of you, bit by bit, until one day, you wake up and don't know who you are anymore.

I felt numb. I felt lost. I felt broken. The things that once brought me joy felt empty. The hope I once clung to felt like a distant memory. I wasn't sure if I would ever truly feel happiness again.

The Pressure and Isolation of Infertility

The pressure we place on ourselves and our bodies is intense. We want so badly what others achieve with ease, yet we must sacrifice everything just for a chance. Infertility demands everything. Our time, our finances, our emotional energy, our sense of self— and yet it offers no guarantees.

It can feel like a punishment, like you're somehow less than others. You would give anything for it to finally be your turn, but no one around you seems to understand the pain that never leaves you.

Infertility is one of the most misunderstood experiences a person can endure. It's not just the physical toll or the endless uncertainty—it's the way the world responds to it.

Instead of compassion, we are met with advice we never asked for. Instead of understanding, we are met with dismissal. Instead of support, we are met with silence.

It feels like I fail every single day. Like I'm being left behind while everyone else moves forward. Like I have no purpose. I am drowning, barely keeping my head above water. Infertility has consumed my identity, and every failure breaks me a little more. Pregnancy announcements make me sad in ways I never expected. I feel more sensitive than ever, overwhelmed by a grief no one else seems to see.

And we are expected to endure it all quietly.

Just because I carry it well doesn't mean it isn't heavy. The world may not see this pain, but that doesn't make it any less real.

The Blame We Shouldn't Carry

Infertility is one of the few medical conditions where blame is placed not just on the body but on the person living in it.

Society, culture, and even our own internal dialogue turn infertility into something personal, something we must have done wrong.

We're told that stress is the problem. That if we just *relaxed* or *stopped trying so hard,* things would magically fall into place. As if infertility is a mindset issue instead of a medical one. As if our own desire is what's standing in the way of what we want most.

We're told that if we lived healthier, ate better, exercised more—but not *too* much—slept more, drank less coffee, took the right supplements, tried acupuncture, or thought *more positively,* we could fix this. As if it was a matter of effort, of willpower, of being *good enough.*

It's infuriating to be blamed for something beyond our control—to carry a heavy pain, only to be met with accusations instead of understanding. And yet, despite all of this, the blame turns inward.

It must be me. It must be my body. It must be something I did, something I didn't do, something I'll never figure out.

But infertility isn't a punishment. It's not a test of worthiness. It's not the result of failing at some invisible standard.

It's a medical condition. But because it's tied so deeply to identity, to the expectations placed upon us, it doesn't feel that way. It feels like a reflection of who we are.

Infertility is so deeply misunderstood because it's often seen as a personal failing rather than what it truly is—a disease. And when the world refuses to recognize it as such, and medical systems continuously fall short in providing the emotional support we need, we end up carrying that blame ourselves.

But infertility isn't our fault. It's not because we're too stressed, too unhealthy, too career-focused, or too *anything*. It's not because of something we did or didn't do.

And no matter how much the world tries to convince us otherwise, we don't have to carry the weight of blame on top of everything else.

We did not cause this. We do not deserve this. Society makes us feel invisible, and we deserve more.

Carrying an Invisible Weight

Infertility becomes a voice in the back of your mind that is impossible to quiet. No one else can hear it. No one can see it. No one truly understands it. But it's there, every day, every month, never fading.

There are moments when you fall apart. And moments when you are so tired of being told how strong you are because being strong is the only choice you have.

With each passing month and each failed cycle, hope starts to dwindle. And when you've been let down so many times before, holding onto hope can feel terrifying.

This path is crushing, and the pain doesn't easily fade. Healing is slow, unpredictable, and often filled with setbacks. But recognizing and validating these emotions is the first step toward healing.

To the person crying in their car on their lunch break. To the person struggling to get through another day. To the person wondering if their time will ever come: I see you. I see you putting on a brave face for a world that doesn't understand the pain you carry through each day.

I spent years convincing myself I was fine too. I was always swallowing the lump in my throat at the grocery store, forcing a smile at work, coming up with reasons to skip events I knew would leave me feeling broken and exhausted.

There were moments I wanted to cry, scream, or hide away. It took me a long time to truly process what was happening internally and years to pick up the pieces.

If you're in this dark place and feel alone in this, know I have felt this weight, and so have many others who have walked this path have felt it too.

Reclaiming Yourself Beyond Infertility

Infertility consumed me. For so long, I looked at my reflection and saw someone I no longer recognized. But one day, I stood there and asked myself, *Who am I beyond infertility?* And slowly, I started searching for that answer.

I started to reclaim parts of myself. It didn't happen overnight, but I began to rediscover the things that made me feel whole outside of this struggle, and you can too.

If today feels impossible, I see you. If you are struggling, I hear you. Today and every day, you matter. Your story matters. Know that it's okay to not always be okay.

There will be days, weeks, and maybe even years where this chapter feels unbearable. But this is one chapter, not your whole story.

Find the people who understand, who will hold space for you, walk with you, and lift you up when you need it most.

This journey is unimaginably hard, so please be kind to yourself.

Infertility isn't just a medical condition; it's a mental health crisis. We need to start talking about it, advocating for better emotional support, and reminding those struggling that they don't have to carry this alone.

You deserve compassion. You deserve care. And most of all, you deserve to be heard.

Prioritize your mental health. Protect your heart. And never forget: You matter. Your pain is real. And no matter how heavy this journey feels, you are never alone.

Your story is not over. There is more to you than this pain, more to your life than this chapter. And one day, you will look back and realize, you survived something unimaginable, and you are still here.

Chapter Eight

Grief Runs Deep

Nothing prepares you for the paralyzing grief of infertility. It's a grief that consumes you, lingering in the spaces between hope and heartbreak.

As someone who has endured infertility and loss, I know how impossible it can feel to put this kind of pain into words. It is grieving what should have been while struggling with what is. It's a grief that stays with you and comes in waves, sometimes years later.

The Grief No One Talks About

I often say infertility is a thief. It doesn't just take away your chance for a baby; it steals who you were. It takes relationships, time, and dreams, leaving behind a version of yourself you barely recognize. The layers of loss run deep, and sometimes, you don't realize how much you are grieving until it consumes you. Infertility grief is mourning every piece of yourself that this journey has taken.

Grief is a big part of infertility and IVF, and no one really prepares you for it. They talk about the cost, the timelines, and the medications, but no one tells you how to cope with the grief that comes with this journey.

Grief is unpredictable. It can be confusing, overwhelming, and hits hardest when you least expect it. You grieve not being able to get pregnant. You grieve lost relationships from people you expected to be in your corner, rooting for you. You grieve the inability to plan for the future because you are trapped in the endless cycle of waiting.

Then there are the countless sacrifices, the ones most will never have to make. Sacrifices that amplify the grief. The financial toll. The trips never taken. The career opportunities put on hold. The moments of joy missed because infertility demands everything. It is consuming, unrelenting, and deeply unfair.

Infertility alters you in ways you never expected. How could it not? It breaks you into pieces, and when you try to put those pieces back together, you realize they'll never fit the same way again.

The grief reaches into every part of your identity. The emotional exhaustion is unlike anything else. The life you once knew feels distant, the person you were feels like a stranger, and all you're left with is the weight of everything you've lost.

This path brings grief that most people could never understand.

It's the grief of having embryos but not knowing if you can afford another cycle or even if, mentally and physically, you can go through it all again for a chance. It's calculating due dates that never come and being reminded every year as these dates pass by. It's experiencing a deep sadness every time your period starts. It's losing months or years of your life that were completely consumed with treatments and trying.

So much of this grief is unspoken, yet it hits harder than expected, sometimes knocking you down completely.

Lost Embryos, Lost Dreams

Lost embryos feel like a piece of you dies. I don't know how to handle the grief or pick up the pieces.

There is a unique pain that comes with embryo loss, one that isn't talked about enough. One thing I wasn't prepared for with IVF was the reality that nothing is guaranteed.

Going into IVF, I wasn't aware of how many eggs wouldn't fertilize, how many embryos wouldn't survive development, what embryo grading meant, or how common a failed cycle was. No one prepared me for the devastating drop-off at every stage.

You endure so much physically and mentally just to reach the point of an egg retrieval during IVF. Then, you wait several agonizing days before receiving your final embryo report. That report is what we all hold our breath for.

I remember waiting for the embryologist to call with updates, my heart stopping every time the phone rang. No one warns you about this waiting period, how powerless you feel, and how there is nothing left to do but hope.

They are your *embabies*. The dreams you have fought so hard for. Each one signifies the possibility of the family you long for.

But what happens when an embryo doesn't survive the thaw? When an embryo doesn't pass genetic testing?

When a cycle fails? When you've done everything right but nothing changes?

The grief is devastating. It is a loss that feels invisible and unbearable. It is sadness, anger, and hopelessness all at once. The weight of it presses down in ways you never imagined. Losing embryos isn't just about the embryos themselves. It's losing time, money, and the future you were desperately hoping for. It's the overwhelming sense of helplessness as everything you worked for slips away.

Embryo loss is profound. A loss rarely acknowledged or understood. But I want you to know that your grief is real. Your pain is valid. And you are not alone.

Embryo loss is the heartbreak of every injection, every appointment, every sacrifice made to create them—only to end without the life you fought so hard to create. It is the weight of so much effort, love, and hope, gone too soon.

And while others may not always understand, I do. Many of us do. And we are grieving alongside you.

When Hope Is Shattered

And then, there are failed cycles. There is the heartbreak of trying again, only to face another devastating setback. The grief that follows makes you question everything.

The hopes and dreams we put into each cycle, the sacrifices we endured, and the strength we needed to push through the pain and fear are gone in a flash. There is nothing quite like going through all of this and having it ripped away by one quick clinical phone call or negative pregnancy test.

One second, you're holding onto hope. The next, it's slipping through your fingers. It's a grief that never gets easier, and no matter how many stories you hear of failed cycles, nothing prepares you for your own. It can feel like your world is collapsing.

I remember one night, sitting on the bathroom floor, staring at another negative test. I felt like the walls were closing in, like I couldn't breathe. The silence was deafening. I wanted to scream, but I had no energy left to even cry. At that moment, I felt completely and utterly hopeless.

Another month, another negative pregnancy test. Another month wasted. Another month of feeling angry, sad, and broken. Another month left wondering, *When will it be my turn?*

Each month that passes feels like a lifetime. You try not to compare your journey to others, but it feels impossible not to. Sometimes, there's jealousy, but usually, it's a profound sadness that things couldn't be easier.

The blame can be overwhelming. The blame we place on ourselves and the blame we sometimes feel from others can be suffocating. *What did I do wrong? How did this happen?* And the more you ask, the more broken you feel.

With each failed cycle, you slowly lose yourself. The version of you that existed before infertility feels more and more distant. The carefree, hopeful version of yourself feels out of reach. And with that distance comes more grief, a quiet and consuming loss for the life and the person you once knew.

I know this path feels impossible. It's quite possibly the hardest thing you have ever endured. Each failed cycle or embryo loss is so painful, yet the world seems to expect you to pick up the pieces and keep going as if nothing happened.

Though many do not validate or understand these types of losses, know that your pain and feelings are real. You did nothing to cause this—you did nothing to deserve this. Sometimes, no matter how much we sacrifice, how hard we try, or how perfectly we follow every step, it still doesn't work, which is the most devastating reality to face, but please know that this is not your fault.

Grief runs deep in this process, and while each loss can feel like a punch in the gut, it's important to recognize and honor this grief.

A failed cycle is loss. Embryo loss is loss.

And every loss deserves to be grieved.

The Weight of Conflicting Emotions

Infertility makes you realize that multiple emotions coexist in ways you never thought possible.

I learned along the way that navigating grief is part of this journey. Shock, denial, guilt, anger, sadness, depression, and eventually, some form of acceptance—it's all there. Some days you feel it all at once. Sometimes it sneaks up on you, but feeling every stage is a necessary part of healing.

In the beginning, I felt a heavy sadness that was hard to understand or explain. I now know it's because infertility changes everything, and I was processing the loss of so many aspects of my life all at once. How could I not grieve that?

Shock and denial were heavy ones to navigate too. My world was collapsing, and it felt like none of this could be real, yet there I was, part of a club I never imagined. There was a lot of anger too. But the hardest part was working toward acceptance. Accepting that infertility was now part of my story. I had to come to terms with it and validate all the complex feelings that came with this life-altering reality.

Once I acknowledged the depths of my grief, I had to figure out how to carry it. How do you begin to heal when your entire world feels broken?

Navigating Grief on Your Own Terms

Grief isn't always visible, but it's there. It's in the hollow feeling you get when you see another pregnancy announcement. It weighs on you with every negative test. It's the sorrow after another embryo transfer doesn't take. But this grief does not define you.

To heal, you have to stop pretending it doesn't hurt. For so long, I told myself I was okay, convincing myself that if I ignored the pain, it would somehow lessen. Despite the emotional, mental, and physical rollercoaster I was experiencing, I kept moving forward as if I was fine. But I have come to realize that pretending to be okay does not protect you. It only postpones the healing process.

Suppressing pain doesn't make it disappear. It lingers beneath the surface, waiting to be acknowledged. Healing requires facing both the good and the painful emotions, allowing yourself to process them rather than bury them. It isn't easy, but neither is carrying the weight of unspoken grief.

Healing is hard. Not healing is harder.

The first and most crucial step in navigating grief is allowing yourself to truly feel it. Grief does not have to be rational or logical. It doesn't follow a timeline, and it cannot be confined to a box. It's okay to be angry, cry, and question why this is happening to you. Give yourself permission to mourn the dreams that never came true and the sadness that comes with every failed cycle or setback. Loss takes many forms, and so does pain.

Your feelings are valid, and they deserve to be honored.

Infertility is an incredibly isolating experience, but you do not have to face it alone. Reaching out for support can make all the difference. That might mean leaning on a partner, confiding in a close friend, joining a support group, or seeking help from a therapist who understands the complexities of infertility grief.

There are communities filled with people who know what you are going through, people who have felt this pain and understand what it's like to carry this every day. Connecting with others can be a powerful reminder that you are not alone in this journey.

Self-care is essential when navigating the emotional weight of infertility. Grief can drain your energy, rob you of joy, and leave you feeling like a shell of yourself. Taking care of your body and mind is essential. That might mean taking a break, engaging in hobbies and activities that spark joy, or simply allowing yourself to rest. Sometimes, self-care is about being gentle with yourself, setting boundaries, giving yourself grace, and letting yourself grieve without judgment.

Building resilience does not mean pretending that everything is okay when it's not. It's about finding ways to stand back up. It's about changing the way you talk to yourself.

It's about accepting that this journey is hard, that it's okay to not be okay, and that moving forward is not the same as moving on. Resilience in infertility is learning to live in the space between hope and heartache, to hold both in your hands without letting one destroy the other.

It's easy to feel like your whole life is wrapped up in infertility, but finding meaning outside of this can be a powerful way to cope. Maybe it's in the small moments that remind you life can still be beautiful, even when it's not the life you planned. Infertility might change your story, but it does not erase the parts of you that make you whole.

I know this chapter is heavy, but so is the one you are living.

The grief of infertility is unlike any other. It's the grief of failed cycles, lost embryos, and dreams that never got the chance to be. It's the sadness of watching your life on hold while the rest of the world moves on. It's losing parts of yourself you never thought you would have to let go of. But in this darkness, there is also a strength that only those who have walked this road can truly understand.

If you are in the depths of infertility grief, know that your pain is real, your struggle is valid, and you are not alone. This journey is brutal, unfair, and often misunderstood. Infertility may shape you, but it does not define you.

Chapter Nine

Your Voice Matters

F or so long, I didn't advocate for the care I deserved. I stayed silent, unsure of how to use my voice in a system that often made me feel powerless. If I knew then what I know now, my journey would have looked entirely different. I imagine many of you feel the same.

That's exactly why I'm here, writing this chapter. It's a chapter dedicated to the power of demanding the care you deserve and advocating for yourself because, for far too long, patients have been forced to navigate a deeply broken system. A system that has left far too many of us in the dark, feeling unheard and unsupported.

Advocating for myself didn't come easily. In fact, it sometimes still doesn't. But I've learned that you must speak up for yourself at the doctor's office, and fertility treatments are no exception.

The cost of infertility is substantial, both literally and figuratively. It often costs you your time, emotional and mental health, dreams, self-worth, relationships, finances, and more. You put yourself through so much, all for just a chance. So yes, you are one hundred percent allowed to ask questions, seek clarity, and demand the care you deserve.

When I began my fertility journey, I hesitated to speak up. The thought of asking questions or expressing concerns filled me with fear. I worried about being seen as difficult or, worse, causing delays in treatment. Waiting is such an excruciating part of this process, and the last thing I wanted was to prolong it. So I kept silent, trusted the care I was receiving, and hoped for the best. And then, one day, I couldn't anymore. I started questioning everything from the care, the recommendations, the lack of support, the critical mistakes, and the direction each cycle seemed to take. I felt confused, heartbroken, and, honestly, angry.

Reflecting on the various decisions and the careless errors, the lack of empathy, and the experiences I had within the walls of the place that should have had my best interests at heart left me baffled.

That's when I realized something: You are allowed to make a big deal about the things that matter to you. You are allowed to ask questions, push for answers, insist on being heard, demand proper treatment, and feel like more than just a number.

Advocating for yourself can feel scary and uncomfortable. Maybe you fear being labeled as *difficult* or worry it might affect your treatment. Maybe you're embarrassed or scared to seem like you don't trust the experts in the room. It can feel like a big deal because, well, it *is* a big deal.

You are standing up for yourself and ensuring you feel confident in your care and the path you are on. Do not underestimate the importance of this. And do not push aside your needs and concerns out of fear or temporary discomfort. This is your life, your journey. You have the right to speak up, especially when something doesn't feel right.

One of my biggest turning points on my journey was realizing there's no such thing as a silly question when it comes to your health. The medications, procedures, and changes your body goes through can feel overwhelming and scary. No one expects you to have all the answers. Whether it's asking why a particular protocol is being recommended, requesting additional testing, or wanting more clarity about medications, you deserve answers.

Doctors and nurses get asked a lot of questions, and chances are, they've heard what you're thinking hundreds of times before. What may feel embarrassing or trivial to you is likely a routine concern they receive.

Like many of you, I turned to Google far too often, trying to find answers on my own instead of bringing my concerns to the people meant to guide me. I learned to remind myself that this is their job. They are there to support, educate, and empower you. And if your care team isn't doing that, it's a sign to consider other options.

Choosing the right clinic is one of the first big decisions you'll make on this journey. It's important to ensure you are with a clinic that truly listens and supports you.

Sadly, not every clinic is created equal. Not every clinic prioritizes patient care. Not every clinic or doctor will be the right fit. Some may dismiss your concerns, rush through appointments, or fail to personalize care to your unique needs. Some may not have as much experience with specific concerns or health conditions that need to be managed.

Over the years, I've heard from countless patients who made the difficult decision to switch clinics after feeling ignored, dismissed, taken advantage of, or stuck in a one-size-fits-all approach.

Know that you have the right to seek care that feels right for you. You don't have to go with the first clinic you speak with or are referred to. You can have consultations with multiple clinics to see what feels like a good fit.

Interview clinics, ask questions, and do your own research.

It took me far too long to understand I wasn't *stuck* with any particular clinic or doctor. You are allowed to get a second or third opinion, change providers, and find a team that genuinely supports you. Whether it's deciding on your first clinic or you're feeling like you're at a crossroads with your current clinic, you have options and say in where to proceed with treatments.

And most importantly, amazing doctors are out there—don't ever settle for less than the care and support you deserve. Choosing the right one is deeply personal, so take your time. Consider location, cost, success rates, policies, patient reviews, and overall care approach. You're putting so much on the line, so make sure you feel confident in your decision.

Practical Ways to Advocate for Yourself

An educated patient is an empowered patient. Ask questions, demand answers, and trust your instincts.

Over the years, I've learned helpful strategies to ensure I'm heard and respected as a patient. These lessons came from many arduous experiences, along with trial and error, but I hope they save you some of the frustration I experienced:

Write everything down. Before any medical appointment, write down your questions, symptoms, or concerns. It's easy to forget things in the moment, especially during emotionally charged discussions. Having questions written down ahead of time ensures everything is addressed. Remember, no question is *silly*, and if it's on your mind, it's worth asking.

Bring a support person. Having a partner, friend, or family member at appointments can provide much value. A second set of ears can help you process information, and you will also have someone to lean on for emotional support. If you can't bring someone with you, ask if it would be okay to record your appointment. This way you can listen back on the appointment to ensure nothing was missed.

Communicate. Don't hesitate to share concerns or what you're feeling. Your care team needs the full picture to provide the best care possible. If something doesn't feel right, trust your instincts, and don't be afraid to consult with another specialist for a second opinion. A fresh perspective can be invaluable.

Do your own research. While the doctor is the fertility expert, no one knows your body better than you do. Educating yourself as a patient can help you feel confident and prepared.It can also assist you in making more informed decisions. I believe everyone should take the time to learn more about their health, treatments, and the path they are on. Research is empowering.

Advocating for yourself requires understanding your unique needs in every aspect: physically, emotionally, mentally, and spiritually. For me, it took navigating multiple diagnoses, including PCOS, endometriosis, autoimmune issues, recurrent implantation failure, and recurrent pregnancy loss to realize that I needed to take control of my journey.

I couldn't keep doing the same treatment over and over again, nor could I rely on anyone else to speak up for me. This realization didn't come easily. There were moments of self-doubt, frustration, and grief. I felt overwhelmed by the pressure to get it right and, occasionally, guilty for questioning my doctors' expertise. But advocating for my care became the best thing I ever did for myself.

Infertility will test you in ways you never imagined, pushing you to your limits and forcing you to fight harder than you ever thought possible. But you have every right to demand the care, respect, and answers you deserve.

Advocating isn't just about asking questions or switching clinics. It's about using your voice, recognizing your worth, and believing in your dreams enough to stand up and say, *I matter.* Because you do.

Chapter Ten

The Club We Never Wanted To Join

Infertility is a club no one ever expects to be part of, yet here we are, bound by an experience that shakes you to your core.

The moment I realized I was part of this club, my world shifted, and suddenly, I was navigating a reality I had never prepared for. It's a battle that changes everything, stays with you forever, and feels impossible to explain to anyone who hasn't lived it.

Infertility will test you in every way possible. It will consume you, making the weight feel unbearable and leaving you questioning if your time will ever come. It will tear you down and force you to rebuild yourself over and over again. It will push you beyond limits you never knew existed, filling your days with tears and your nights with worry.

It's lying awake at 3 a.m., staring at the ceiling, calculating dates, injections, and timelines over and over. It's the sadness, anger, and heartache every time someone asks, *Do you have kids?* It's forcing a smile and pretending far too often that you're okay when you're breaking inside. It's the deep, aching loneliness, even in a crowded room.

But if there's one thing that makes any of this more bearable, it's the strength we find in each other. Community is what holds us up when we feel like we're falling, reminding us that we're never truly alone with any of this—the anger, grief, waiting, dread, or fear.

The Strength in Community

There was a time where I spent countless nights searching for answers, convinced no one understood my pain. But when I started sharing my story and found others walking this same path, I realized I wasn't alone, and that changed everything.

The IVF Warrior wasn't just about creating a space to vent frustrations. I was exhausted from navigating a broken system that felt clinical and confusing. Worn down by a weight no one around me seemed to understand. Drained by the thoughts that consumed me every day.

I know firsthand the continuous daily challenges faced, the loneliness that can take over, and the confusion of doing this alone, and I needed to help change this. Without community, I felt broken, lost, and alone.

I felt as though the overwhelming thoughts and emotions I felt weren't common, which added to an already isolating experience. I didn't want others to feel the way I did.

When you're going through infertility, it's not just a diagnosis—it affects every part of your existence. It impacts your mental, physical, and emotional health, sometimes all at once. It's a disease that affects millions worldwide, yet because of the silence, it can feel so lonely.

Being part of a community that truly understands can make the toughest days feel a little lighter. It validates your feelings and struggles, reminding you that there is no right or wrong way to navigate this journey. Whether it's cheering each other on, sitting in the hard together, grieving losses, or simply listening without judgment, community creates a space unlike any other.

And as much as it's about supporting each other, it's also about connection and discovering strength we didn't always know we had.

Community is built on kindness and reminders like, *Your feelings are valid* and *Your story matters.*

These simple messages can be the encouragement you need on the hardest days, offering reassurance that your pain is real and your experience matters.

Infertility can be so heavy, but community is a reminder that you're part of something bigger. People who understand this shared, painful experience are rooting for you.

Breaking the Silence

Sharing our struggles with others can come with a lot of thoughts and emotions. Putting your experience into words, whether spoken, written, or shared, can make it feel even more real. And with that comes both fear and healing. I know this because it took me a while to feel comfortable enough to open up about my journey.

When I first started sharing, I was flooded with emotion and didn't know if I could find the right words. I remember sitting with my phone, fingers hovering over the keyboard, deleting and retyping my words, terrified of what people might say. What if they didn't get it? What if they minimized my pain? What if no one cared? But in the end, I hit "post," and I held my breath.

What happened next was something I never expected.

Within minutes, the notifications started. Comments. Messages. Stories from people I had never met but who understood exactly what I was going through. People who had also felt the gut-wrenching pain of another failed cycle, the exhaustion of endless waiting, the heartbreak of feeling left behind and broken.

Some had been carrying their pain in silence for years, afraid to say the words out loud. Others had never met someone who truly understood, someone who didn't offer false hope or dismissive reassurances, but who simply said, *Me too.*

I read messages from people in the thick of it who were drowning in grief and searching for someone who could put their pain into words. I read stories from those who had been fighting for years. I saw comments from people who had been through it all and came out the other side, carrying the weight of what it took to get there.

And in those stories, I saw pieces of my own.

It was the first time I truly understood the power of community, the power of simply being seen. The moment I started opening up, it felt like a weight had been lifted.

I had spent so long feeling alone in my grief, convinced that no one could possibly understand what I was going through. But suddenly, I wasn't holding this all on my own. I was speaking to people who lived with this too.

It was healing for me, but even more than that, I realized how much it could help others who might be struggling in silence. The simple act of sharing my story created space for others to share theirs, for people to finally feel seen in a world that so often ignores this kind of pain.

That was the moment everything changed.

Finding Your Voice and Your People

I remember the first time I opened up to my closest friend, I was terrified. I worried they wouldn't understand, or worse, that they would dismiss my pain. But I learned that the right people will listen, and having even one person who truly gets it can make all the difference. Opening up can be scary, but it can also be incredibly freeing.

If you're unsure how to share your story, start small. A single message, a conversation with a trusted friend, or even allowing yourself to journal your emotions can help. Every step matters.

Other options to find connection and community are available too.

Joining a local or online support group can also be helpful. These spaces offer connection with others who truly understand, providing a sense of belonging and validation in an otherwise isolating experience.

A therapist, especially one familiar with infertility, can also provide a safe space to process your emotions while offering coping tools and strategies tailored to your journey.

Many people also find community on social media, where there are others sharing similar journeys. If you aren't ready to share your face or name, know that creating an anonymous account still allows you to connect with fertility sites like The IVF Warrior, along with those on this path.

No matter how you choose to navigate this, the key is knowing that support is there when you need it. You don't have to go through this alone, and there is no *right* way to seek support.

Also know that this, right here, is a community. These pages, these words, are a place to return to whenever you need to feel seen, validated, and understood.

You Are Not Alone

I know the weight of waiting. The unbearable silence. The feeling that everyone else is moving forward while you stand still. I know the way grief sneaks up on you, the way hope feels dangerous, and the way you brace yourself for yet another heartbreak.

But I also know this: You are not broken. You are not alone. And you do not have to carry this by yourself.

Infertility makes you feel like you're walking this path alone, but you're not. There's an entire community of people who see you, hear you, and carry this weight alongside you.

To those in the wait, I see you. I know the heartache of wondering when or if it will ever be your turn. The fear that lingers with every passing month. The pain of feeling like you're behind. The grief that is silent but deafening.

I know this is the heaviest, most misunderstood experience, but I hope these words remind you that you are not broken. You are not failing. You are navigating something unimaginably hard.

Infertility can feel like the worst club with the best members. None of us chose this, but we carry each other through. In the hardest moments, we stand beside one another, offering strength and reminding each other that even in the darkest times, we are never truly alone.

Your story is still being written. This chapter may be filled with pain, uncertainty, and waiting, but it is not the whole story. However this unfolds, you are still here. And that is enough.

Infertility may have changed you, but it will never define you. You are so much more than this struggle. And no matter what happens next, you will find your way forward.

And even now, even here, there is still hope. Hope in the strength you have shown. Hope in the community that surrounds you. Hope in the possibility of joy beyond this pain. You are not alone. And you are not without hope.

Conclusion

Infertility is a journey that changes you. It challenges your sense of self, tests your relationships, and forces you to navigate emotions and conversations that most people will never have to face. It makes you question everything—your body, your future, your strength, your trust in what you once believed was certain.

Infertility is not just about trying to have a baby. It's about feeling powerless in a world that tells you to just *trust the process.* It's about making impossible choices that come with no guarantees. It's about learning to hold grief and hope in the same breath, to survive heartbreak after heartbreak while still daring to dream of something more.

If there's one thing I hope you take away from these pages, it's this: you are not alone.

Infertility can feel isolating, like an experience that separates you from the rest of the world, but you are not the only one walking this path. So many of us have been where you are. The grief, the frustration, the exhaustion, the longing—you are not alone in any of it. Your pain is valid. Your emotions are real. Your story matters.

You Are Not Defined by This Struggle

Infertility may change the way you see yourself, your relationships, and even the world around you, but it does not define you. You are not broken because of this. You are not less worthy. You are not failing.

This journey forces you to make impossible decisions and ask yourself questions you never thought you'd have to answer. *How much more can I take? How far do I go? When do I stop?* It pushes you to the edge of your emotional limits, only to ask you to keep going. It requires you to find strength in moments of despair and redefine hope after every setback. It demands that you learn to carry grief in a way no one ever prepared you for.

But no matter how much infertility has changed you, it will never take away who you are at your core. You are still you. You are still worthy. You are still whole, even if this journey has made you feel otherwise.

The Power in Your Story

I never expected infertility to become such a defining part of my life, but it has shaped me in ways I never could have imagined. It has broken me and rebuilt me. It has made me more resilient, more compassionate, and more aware of the invisible struggles people carry. It has shown me that pain and strength can exist in the same space, that grief and hope are not opposites but intertwined.

Infertility will change you in ways you never thought possible. But it will also reveal strengths you never knew you had.

I hope you see that strength within yourself too.

Wherever You Are, Your Journey Is Valid

As you move forward, whether you're still in the trenches of infertility, stepping into a new path, or trying to re-claim pieces of yourself after years of fighting, know this: There is no right or wrong way to do this. Your journey is yours alone, and whatever decisions you make, whether you continue, pause, stop, or shift directions, are valid. Healing will take time. It's okay to not always be okay. It's okay to still feel the weight of this, no matter where you are now.

Give yourself grace. And allow yourself to grieve.

Finding Joy Again

One of the hardest lessons infertility teaches is learning to sit with the unknown. To exist in a space where control is an illusion and certainty is out of reach. But within that uncertainty, there is still a life to be lived.

Infertility doesn't mean you have to live in sadness forever. It doesn't mean your life has to be defined by loss. You are allowed to find joy in the in-between moments. You are allowed to laugh, to dream, to move forward, not because you've *let go* or *moved on,* but because you deserve happiness, no matter how your story unfolds.

Honoring Your Strength

Throughout these chapters, we've explored the physical, emotional, and mental toll infertility takes, the silent battles fought daily, and the strength it requires to keep moving forward despite the continuous heartbreak.

We talk so much about the pain of infertility, but I also want to acknowledge your quiet moments of courage, the small victories that deserve to be recognized.

Every time you showed up for another appointment, braced yourself for another needle, or held onto hope even when you felt like giving up—that was strength. Every time you allowed yourself to cry, to feel, to sit in your grief—that was resilience.Every time you advocated for yourself, asked questions, sought support—that was power.

You may not always see it, but you are stronger than you realize.

Your Story Isn't Over

The conversation about infertility is far from over. And neither is your story.

I hope this book has provided comfort, validation, and a sense of understanding in a world that often overlooks the depth of this struggle. I hope it has reminded you that no matter where you are in your journey, you are seen, you are heard, and you are never alone.

You have the right to advocate for yourself, set boundaries, protect your heart, and make decisions that align with what is best for you.

Your pain is real. But so is your power.

Final Words to Carry With You

If there's anything I want you to carry with you after closing this book, it's the knowledge that:

Infertility doesn't define you.

You are not alone.

Your voice matters.

Your experience matters.

You matter.

So keep advocating. Keep hoping. Keep believing in yourself.

Because no matter where this journey takes you, you are already enough.

More Than Infertility

And lastly, remember this: Infertility may be part of your story, but it is not your whole story.

You are more than this. You are worthy of love. You are worthy of joy. And you are worthy of a life that is filled with happiness, no matter how your story unfolds.

Dear Warrior: Words for the Moments That Feel Impossible

Infertility is heavy, isolating, and on some days, it feels like too much to carry.

These letters are for those days.

For the days when hope feels distant. For the moments when the weight of waiting, uncertainty, and exhaustion feel too heavy to carry. For when Mother's Day arrives like a quiet storm, or when well-meaning words from friends and family only deepen the ache.

I want you to have something to hold onto in those moments.

Whether you need reassurance that your feelings are valid, comfort on a day that feels impossible, or words to help the people in your life better understand this journey, these letters are here for you. To remind you that you are seen. That you are not broken. That even in the hardest moments, you are never alone.

Take what you need. Share what helps. Return to these words when the weight feels too heavy. And please, never forget: you are worthy of love, care, and understanding, always.

***

A Letter for Your Hardest Days

Dear Warrior,

I know.

I know how heavy this feels. How unfair. How cruel. How impossible.

I know that today, hope feels out of reach. That you're exhausted from holding on, from trying, from convincing yourself to keep going when all you want to do is collapse under the weight of it all.

I know that no one around you truly understands. That the world keeps moving forward while you're stuck in this endless cycle of heartbreak, disappointment, and waiting. That no matter how much you try to explain, your pain feels invisible. That the people who love you don't always know how to show up, and maybe today, it feels like you have no one at all.

I know that infertility isn't just about struggling to have a baby. It's about feeling like you've lost control of your own life. It's about sacrificing time, money, relationships, and pieces of yourself you never imagined losing. It's about waking up every day with the same aching question of when or if this will ever change.

I know you don't feel strong. I know you're exhausted from having to be strong all the time. Of being told how resilient you are when all you want is for this to be easier. I know it feels like you have lost your way, like the person you used to be is slipping further away with each setback, loss, and impossible decision you have to make.

I know that today, you feel like a failure, like your body has let you down in ways that are impossible to put into words. Like no matter how much you fight, it's never enough. Like the weight of this grief is too much to bear.

But please, hear me when I say this.

You are not broken. You are not weak. You are not failing.

You are surviving something that's unimaginable, something that's isolating, consuming, and relentless. Even when you feel like you're drowning, you keep going. Even when you feel like you have nothing left, you're still here. And that is strength in its purest form.

I know it doesn't feel like it right now, but this moment, this crushing and unbearable moment, is not forever.

You don't have to fix it today. You don't have to find the silver lining or force yourself to believe in hope. You don't have to pretend to be okay when you're not.

Because sometimes, things just suck. Sometimes, life is unfair, and it's okay to say that. It's okay to be angry. It's okay to scream, to cry, to fall apart. It's okay to wonder why this is happening to you.

But please, don't believe the lie that you are alone in this.

Because I am here.

I am here in the moments when no one else seems to be. I am here when the world feels like it's caving in around you. I am here when the negative tests pile up, when another cycle fails, when you're too numb to cry, too exhausted to hope, and too worn down to believe this will ever change.

I am here, sitting with you in this pain. Holding space for the weight of what you're carrying. And I won't tell you to just stay positive, that everything happens for a reason, or that it will all make sense someday. Because right now, that's not what you need.

What you need is for someone to say: I see you. I know how much this hurts. And I won't let you sit in this darkness alone.

So if today feels unbearable, if you're questioning every-thing, if you don't know where to turn, let this letter re-mind you that you don't have to carry this by yourself.

You are worthy of love and support, even on the days when you feel like you have nothing left to give.

You are more than your worst day.

And you are not alone.

With all my love,

Someone who has been where you are and is standing with you.

***

To Those in the Wait on Mother's Day

To Those in the Wait on Mother's Day,

I see you.

I see the pain you carry, the silent ache that lingers in your heart, and the unbearable weight of another Mother's Day spent waiting. I know how deeply you long for the day when this holiday will feel different. When the grief won't consume you. When you won't have to hold back tears as you smile through the celebrations of others.

I know this day is one of the hardest.

It's a day filled with reminders of what you don't have, of what you're still fighting for, of how unfair this journey has been. It's the social media posts, the commercials, the greeting cards in every store, the well-meaning but painful words of others. It's another year of wondering when it will finally be your turn.

I know you thought this Mother's Day would be different. That maybe this year, you'd be holding your baby instead of holding back tears. That maybe, for once, this day wouldn't feel so isolating.

I know it hurts.

I know that as you scroll past pregnancy announcements and Mother's Day tributes, your heart aches for the moment that you will be celebrated too. I know that it stings in a way that's impossible to explain.

I know that no matter how strong you are, today might break you.

I know that some will tell you to stay hopeful or just be grateful for what you have. But what they don't understand is that you can be grateful for your life and still grieve what is missing. You can be hopeful and heartbroken at the same time.

I want you to know that your pain is real. Your grief is valid. And it's okay to not be okay.

You don't have to push through. You don't have to celebrate. You don't have to pretend this day isn't excruciating just to make others more comfortable. It's okay to step away, protect your heart, and do whatever you need to do to get through.

If you want to stay off social media, do it.If you need to decline invitations, that's okay.If you need to cry, let yourself.If you want to scream about how unfair this is, you have every right to.

Because this is unfair. This is cruel. This is a grief that is invisible to so many, yet it consumes every part of you.

And I know that today, that grief might feel heavier than ever.

But I want you to know this. You are not alone.

So many of us are sitting in this pain together, navigating this same impossible day, longing for the moment when it won't hurt quite as much. When we, too, will be seen, acknowledged, and celebrated.

To the one still waiting, still hoping, still aching for the day when this pain will ease, I see you.

To the one who is grieving a baby in their heart but not in their arms, I honor you.

To the one wondering when it will finally be their turn, you are not forgotten.

To the one who doesn't know what their future holds, you are not alone.

You are a mother in the deepest, most unrecognized way. A mother in the love you already have, in the fight you continue to endure, in the dreams that live inside you.

And no matter how this day unfolds, you matter.

Your story matters.

Your pain matters.

And even if the world doesn't acknowledge it today, I do.

With all my love,

Someone who carries this pain with you.

***

Dear Friends and Family

Dear Friends and Family,

Infertility is one of the most devastating experiences a person can go through.

Just because I look fine doesn't mean I'm not hurting. Just because I don't always talk about it doesn't mean I'm not struggling. And just because I carry it well doesn't mean it isn't heavy.

Infertility is a thief. It consumes you, reshaping your world, straining relationships, and changing the person you once were. It's a voice that never fades. A silent pain buried deep within your soul.

Unless you've lived it, you can't possibly understand infertility. It's impossible to grasp the weight of uncertainty, the emotional toll of hope and heartbreak, and the grief of what should have been. I don't expect you to have the right words. I don't expect you to fix this. But what I do hope for is compassion. Understanding. The space to grieve this loss without judgment.

Because that's what infertility is—a grief that runs deep. A grief that lingers in every conversation, experience, and interaction. A grief that reshapes your entire world.

Infertility is more than struggling to have a baby. It's about feeling powerless, like nothing is in my control. It's being angry at my body for failing me. It's watching my dreams slip further away, feeling completely out of reach. It's living in a relentless cycle of uncertainty, making sacrifices most will never have to make, all for a chance. It's enduring month after month, year after year, trapped between hope and despair. It's feeling behind as friends and family move forward with their lives, while my life stands still. It's grieving something no one around me sees, and it's unbearably lonely.

Infertility isn't just a physical struggle. It's an emotional and mental battle that is often far more difficult to endure. The injections, procedures, and medications are hard, but the toll it takes on your mind is even harder. It's the way infertility consumes your thoughts from the moment you wake up to the moment you fall asleep.

It's the fear of the unknown, the crushing anxiety of waiting, and the exhaustion of constantly hoping, only to be disappointed. It's feeling like you have no control over your body, your future, or the life you once envisioned. The mental weight of infertility is relentless, isolating, and invisible to the outside world, making it even harder to carry. While the physical pain fades, the emotional scars remain, shaping the way you see yourself, your relationships, and the world around you.

I hear the comments. *Just relax. It will happen when you stop trying. Have you thought about adoption? At least you can sleep in.* I know you mean well, but some words hurt more than they help. Saying *Just stop stressing* or *Take a vacation* doesn't make me feel better. It makes me feel dismissed. Being overly optimistic doesn't make me feel better either. Telling me to *just stay positive* only makes me feel like my pain is being ignored. Infertility is a medical disease, not something I can fix by thinking differently.

Would you tell someone grieving a loss that everything happens for a reason? Would you tell someone in pain that they just need to stay positive? Infertility is often met with dismissive comments that no other medical condition would be. It's hard not to feel broken and to blame yourself, and the way society treats this disease doesn't help.

Please think before you speak. I don't need silver linings. I don't need my pain minimized or reframed as a lesson in patience. Infertility isn't a mindset problem, and optimism won't change my reality. It's something I have to live with every single day.

What I need is support. Understanding. Acknowledgment of how devastating this is.

Please check in on me. A simple *I'm thinking of you* means more than you know. Even if I don't always respond, knowing I'm not forgotten in this struggle makes a difference. Please continue to invite me. Don't exclude me. I may not always feel up to socializing, but feeling left out hurts even more. Let me decide what I can handle.

Please understand that this journey is all-consuming. Fertility treatments aren't just physically exhausting. They take over my entire life. The medications, the doctor's appointments, the waiting, the uncertainty. It's a full-time job with no guarantee of success.

Please allow me to share on my own terms. I know you care, and I know you want to be there for me. But infertility is deeply personal, and sometimes I need time to process before I share. There are moments I want to talk and moments I just want to be. Please don't push for updates, and please don't take it personally if I don't have the energy to explain every step. I'll give an update when I'm ready.

Some situations are harder than others. Baby showers, pregnancy announcements, holidays, and family gatherings filled with well-meaning questions like, *When are you having kids?* are painful. These moments are triggering and difficult to endure, yet I'm expected to smile, celebrate, and push my feelings aside. Please try to recognize how deeply unfair and hurtful that is. My feelings are valid.

Know that infertility doesn't just go away. No matter the outcome, it will always be a part of me. The trauma, the loss, and the grief don't simply disappear. This experience stays with you forever, and it's something no one seems to understand. It's the cruelest kind of grief, one that no one acknowledges, yet it never stops hurting.

Each failed cycle is soul-crushing. Each month feels like another piece of me breaks. It's impossible to explain this grief unless you've experienced it. Infertility is suffocating. It's a silent, unseen heartbreak that we carry while the world expects us to keep functioning as if we're not falling apart inside. But silence is heavy, and pretending to be okay is exhausting.

You may never fully understand what I'm going through, but my hope is that this letter helps you see that infertility is so much more than what meets the eye.

I need you to understand that this is my life, my journey, and the choices I make are mine alone.

I don't need you to know every medical term, procedure, or decision I make. I just need you to understand that this is one of the hardest things I will ever go through. Just because you can't see the weight of it doesn't mean it isn't there.

I need you to see that this is real, that it's painful, and that your support matters more than you may ever realize. I need you to stand beside me, not just for the happy endings but for the moments when I feel like I may never get one.

Because this isn't just a hard chapter in my life.

This is my life.

I know it's not easy to watch someone you love go through this, but your support means everything. I don't need perfect words. I don't need you to fix it.

I just need you to be here.

To acknowledge my pain. To sit with me in the hard moments without trying to rush me through them. To walk beside me, even when you don't know what to say.

Infertility will test me in ways I never imagined, but knowing I have people who stand beside me, people who don't try to dismiss, minimize, or fix my pain, makes all the difference.

Thank you for being here.

With love, in the hope that you truly see me.

Acknowledgements

This book exists because of the countless voices that have been silenced, the emotions too heavy to share, and the stories buried beneath grief. To every person who has walked this path, felt unseen, or carried the unbearable weight of infertility in silence, this is for you.

To the infertility community, my fellow warriors, the ones who have fought, endured, and survived the unimaginable—you have given me purpose, and you have given each other hope. Your strength, vulnerability, and willingness to share the hardest parts of your life have shaped this book in ways I cannot express.

To those who have shared their truth with me, who have trusted me with their pain, and who have reminded me that none of us are ever truly alone—your words, your resilience, and your unspoken battles live within these pages.

To my publishing team, thank you for taking a chance on me, for recognizing the urgency of amplifying conversations about infertility, and for believing in the work I do at *The IVF Warrior*. Your support has meant everything. Each of you has guided me, motivated me, and helped me bring this book to life in a way that feels true, not just to me but to all of us who have lived this reality. Writing this book was one of the most emotionally difficult projects of my life, and you allowed me to do it in a way that was my own. For that, I am forever grateful.

I wasn't prepared for how deeply this process would affect me. There were tears, frustration, reflection, sadness, and hope poured into every word. Talking about the unspoken aspects of infertility, putting into words what so many suffer in silence, was heavier than I anticipated. I wasn't sure if I would be able to fully capture the depths of it all, but I knew I had to try. I wanted people to feel, relate, and see themselves in these pages. I wanted to give these emotions the justice they deserve. I have spent years trying to speak on the hard parts, but I needed a space to say more because there is so much more to infertility than what the world sees.

To every person who has ever supported *The IVF Warrior*, thank you. To the thousands of medical professionals who share our mission with your patients, to the millions who turn to our platform for information, validation, and support, and to the incredible friends I've met through our shared pain, you have helped create a space where no one has to feel alone in this journey.

To my friends and family, the ones who never turned away. I know this journey may not be one you have experienced firsthand, and I'm sure there were words within these pages that surprised you. But I hope, through them, you can begin to understand just how life-changing this experience was, the weight it carried, the way it shaped me, and the motivation behind everything I do.

M, You kept hope alive when it felt lost. You saw what others couldn't. You understood that I didn't need the perfect words, just someone to acknowledge how hard this was. Your presence spoke volumes in ways I can never fully express. I am forever thankful for you and the love and support you have always provided me.

To my parents. Mom, thank you for always supporting me, cheering me on, and being there when I need you. I am so grateful for you. Dad, you have always believed in me and made sure I knew it. I'm so thankful for the time we've had to grow together. I love you both.

RLK, I love you more than words could ever express. All I've ever wanted is for you to know, without a doubt, that you are loved unconditionally. You are the motivation behind everything I do. The reason I continue to push, to speak up, and to fight for the millions struggling. Even when it's hard. Even when it's uncomfortable. Even when it's scary. You have unknowingly helped so many simply by existing. You are the light in this story.

To Shane, my partner. We have been through so much, and through it all, you have loved me so fiercely. Thank you for standing by me through the darkest moments, for holding space when there were no words. Your support and love mean more than you will ever know. You believed in me when I didn't believe in myself, lifted me when I felt I had nothing left to give, wiped my tears more times than I can count, and reminded me of my strength when I felt lost.

You stood beside me through every heartbreak, every set-back, and every moment when I wasn't sure I could keep going. Because of you, hope was never truly lost. You have been my biggest fan from the very beginning—with *The IVF Warrior*, with this book, and in all the in-between moments, dreams, and ideas. I am endlessly grateful for you and the life we fought so hard to build together.

And finally, to you, the reader holding these pages. Whether you're in the thick of this battle, on the other side, or simply trying to understand, thank you for being here. Thank you for listening to the words that have so often gone unspoken.

I have been where you are. I have sat in the waiting, felt the ache of uncertainty, and carried the weight of grief that no one else could see. I know how isolating this journey can be, how heavy it feels, and how hard it is to hold onto hope when it keeps slipping through your hands.

May this book remind you that your pain is real, your grief is valid, and your voice, whether spoken or unspoken, deserves to be heard.

With all my heart,

Cheryl